The Affordable Care Act

Long-term care in the United States and other countries suffers multiple problems. Many people find it difficult to afford the high costs of services. Care quality is often suboptimal; so too is care coordination, particularly amongst those receiving services paid for by multiple public programs. Recruitment and retention of a well-trained, stable workforce is a challenge as well.

The policy debate leading up to the Patient Protection and Affordable Care Act (ACA) drew attention to prevailing deficiencies in the way long-term care is delivered, regulated, and financed in the United States. This collection reviews what was accomplished by the legislation and what still remains to be done. Just how effective is the ACA likely to be in addressing the challenges plaguing the long-term care sector? Did it result in meaningful change or make little impact? This book answers these questions, drawing contributions from among the most eminent long-term care experts in the United States.

This book was originally published as a special issue of the *Journal of Aging & Social Policy*.

Edward Alan Miller, PhD, M.P.A., is an Associate Professor of Gerontology & Public Policy and Fellow of the Gerontologist Institute at the McCormack Graduate School for Policy & Global Studies at the University of Massachusetts Boston, USA. He is also Adjunct Associate Professor of Health Services, Policy & Practice, at Brown University, USA. His research focuses on understanding the determinants and effects of federal and state policies affecting vulnerable populations. He coauthored the book, *Digital Medicine: Health Care in the Internet Era* (Brookings Institution Press, 2009).

The Affordable Care Act

Advancing Long-Term Care Policy in the United States

Edited by
Edward Alan Miller

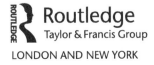
Routledge
Taylor & Francis Group

LONDON AND NEW YORK

First published 2013
by Routledge
2 Park Square, Milton Park, Abingdon, Oxon, OX14 4RN

Simultaneously published in the USA and Canada
by Routledge
711 Third Avenue, New York, NY 10017

First issued in paperback 2017

Routledge is an imprint of the Taylor & Francis Group, an informa business

British Library Cataloguing in Publication Data
A catalogue record for this book is available from the British Library

Typeset in Times New Roman
by Taylor & Francis Books

Publisher's Note
The publisher would like to make readers aware that the chapters in this book may be referred to as articles as they are identical to the articles published in the special issue. The publisher accepts responsibility for any inconsistencies that may have arisen in the course of preparing this volume for print.

ISBN 13: 978-1-138-11567-5 (pbk)
ISBN 13: 978-0-415-63489-2 (hbk)

Contents

v

Citation Information

The following chapters were originally published in the *Journal of Aging & Social Policy*, volume 24, issue 2 (April-June 2012). When citing this material, please use the original page numbering for each article, as follows:

Notes on Contributors

Natasha Bryant, MA, is Senior Research Associate at the LeadingAge Center for Applied Research, Washington, District of Columbia, USA.

Rachel B. Edwards, BA, is a Doctoral Student in the Department of Health Policy and Management at the School of Rural Public Health, Texas A&M Health Science Center, College Station, Texas, USA.

David C. Grabowski, PhD, is Associate Professor in the Department of Health Care Policy at Harvard Medical School, Boston, Massachusetts, USA.

Charlene Harrington, PhD, is Professor in the Department of Social and Behavioral Sciences at the University of California, San Francisco, California, USA.

Catherine Hawes, PhD, is Regents Professor in the Department of Health Policy and Management at the School of Rural Public Health, Texas A&M Health Science Center, College Station, Texas, USA.

H. Stephen Kaye, PhD, is Professor in the Institute for Health and Aging at the University of California, San Francisco, California, USA.

Mitchell LaPlante, PhD, is Professor in the Institute for Health and Aging at the University of California, San Francisco, California, USA.

Mark R. Meiners, PhD is Professor of Health Administration and Policy at George Mason University, Fairfax, Virginia, USA.

Edward Alan Miller, PhD, M.P.A., is an Associate Professor of Gerontology and Public Policy and Fellow of the Gerontologist Institute at the McCormack Graduate School for Policy and Global Studies at the University of Massachusetts Boston, USA. He is also Adjunct Associate Professor of Health Services, Policy & Practice, at Brown University, USA.

Marilyn Moon, PhD, is Senior Vice President of the American Institutes for Research, Silver Spring, Maryland, USA.

Darcy M. Moudouni, PhD, is Assistant Research Scientist in the Department of Health Policy and Management, at the School of Rural Public Health, Texas A&M Health Science Center, College Station, Texas, USA.

Pamela Nadash, PhD, is Assistant Professor of Gerontology, and Fellow of the Gerontology Institute, at the University of Massachusetts Boston, Boston, Massachusetts, USA.

Terence Ng, JD, MA, is Senior Research Analyst for the Department of Social and Behavioral Sciences at the University of California, San Francisco, California, USA.

Charles D. Phillips, PhD, MPH, is Regents Professor in the Department of Health Policy and Management, at the School of Rural Public Health, Texas A&M Health Science Center, College Station, Texas, USA.

Robyn I. Stone, DrPH, is Executive Director at the LeadingAge Center for Applied Research, Washington, District of Columbia, USA.

William G. Weissert, PhD, is Professor at Florida State University, and Director of Masters of Public Health. He is Faculty Associate for the Pepper Institute on Aging & Public Policy at Florida State University, Tallahassee, Florida, USA, and Professor Emeritus at the University of Michigan, Ann Arbor, Michigan, USA.

Joshua M. Wiener, PhD, is Distinguished Fellow and Program Director for Aging, Disability, and Long-Term Care at RTI International, Washington, District of Columbia, USA.

INTRODUCTION

The Affordable Care Act and Long-Term Care: Comprehensive Reform or Just Tinkering Around the Edges?

EDWARD ALAN MILLER, PhD, MPA

Associate Professor of Gerontology and Public Policy, and Fellow, Gerontology Institute, University of Massachusetts Boston, Boston, Massachusetts, USA

The Patient Protection and Affordable Care Act (ACA) includes several provisions that aim to improve prevailing deficiencies in

---

Edward Alan Miller, PhD, MPA, is an associate professor of gerontology and public policy and fellow at the Gerontology Institute, University of Massachusetts Boston. After receiving his PhD in 2003 in Political Science and Health Services Organization & Policy from the University of Michigan, Dr. Miller completed a postdoctoral fellowship in the Department of Epidemiology and Public Health at Yale University. He also holds an AB and MPA from Cornell University and has spent time in New Zealand as a Fulbright scholar and at the Congressional Research Service as a social policy analyst. Dr. Miller's research focuses on understanding the determinants and effects of federal and state policies affecting vulnerable populations, including the frail and disabled elderly, mentally ill, and veterans. His specializations include aging and long-term care, telemedicine and e-health, intergovernmental relations, and program implementation and evaluation. He has published nearly 80 peer-reviewed journal articles. Recent publications have appeared in *The Gerontologist, American Journal of Public Health, Medical Care Research & Review, Journal of Health Politics, Policy, & Law, Review of Policy Research, Health Services Research, International Journal of Geriatric Psychiatry,* and *Journal of Aging & Social Policy*. He organized the August 2010 special issue of *Medical Care Research & Review* on long-term care policy development. He coauthored the book *Digital Medicine: Health Care in the Internet Era,* which was published by Brookings Institution Press in 2009. Dr. Miller is a member of the editorial boards of *The Gerontologist, Journal of Aging & Social Policy, Journal of Health Politics, Policy, & Law, and World Medical & Health Policy*. He was formerly an assistant professor of public policy, political science, and community health at Brown University, where he is now an adjunct associate professor of health services, policy, and practice.

the nation's long-term care system. But just how effective is the ACA likely to be in addressing these challenges? Will it result in meaningful or marginal reform? This special issue of Journal of Aging & Social Policy *seeks to answer these questions. The most prominent long-term care provision is the now-suspended Community Living Assistance Services and Supports Act. Others include incentives and options for expanding home- and community-based care, a number of research and demonstration projects in the areas of chronic care coordination and the dually eligible, and nursing home quality reforms. There are also elements that seek to improve workforce recruitment and retention, in addition to benefit improvements and spending reductions under Medicare. This article reviews the basic problems plaguing the long-term care sector and the provisions within the ACA meant to address them. It also includes a brief overview of issue content.*

INTRODUCTION

Nearly 13 million Americans need long term services and supports, including 10.9 million community residents and 1.8 million individuals residing in nursing homes (Kaye, Harrington, & LaPlante, 2010). Approximately half of community residents are younger than 65; most (92%) receive unpaid care, comparatively few (13%) paid assistance. Since the prevalence of functional and cognitive impairment increases with age, the demand for long-term care (LTC) will grow with the aging population. Between 2008 and 2050, the number of Americans aged 65 years or older will more than double, from 38.9 to 88.5 million, while the number aged 85 years or older triples, from 5.7 to 19.0 million (Federal Interagency Forum on Aging Related Statistics, 2010). Given prevailing deficiencies caring for the current population of elders, general consensus exists that the nation is far from ready to care for the next, much larger generation in need (Miller, Mor, & Clark, 2010; Wiener, Freiman, & Brown, 2007). The Patient Protection and Affordable Care Act (ACA) (P.L. 111–148) includes several provisions that may serve as the basis for meeting current and future challenges in this area.

The ACA was signed into law by President Obama on March 23, 2010. It was subsequently modified with enactment of the Health Care and Education Reconciliation Act on March 30, 2010. Although receiving little notice in light of the broader effort to expand access to basic health insurance coverage for the nation's uninsured population (Miller, 2011), the impact of the ACA on LTC has received more attention recently. This is largely the result of the Obama Administration's decision to abandon implementation of the Community Living Assistance Services and Supports (CLASS) Act, a provision within the ACA that would have established a national, federally administered voluntary LTC insurance program. The administration concluded that it had limited legal authority to make unilateral changes that addressed fatal flaws in the program's basic design and, as such, could not ensure 75 years of financial solvency as required by the law (Gleckman, 2011). It also recognized that the prevailing partisan political dynamic precluded shepherding the necessary changes that addressed these flaws through Congress. But the CLASS Act is not the entire story. The ACA includes a number of other provisions meant to address extant deficiencies in the LTC sector, including with respect to home- and community-based services (HCBS), care coordination, nursing home quality, and caregiving. This special issue of the *Journal of Aging & Social Policy* analyzes elements of the ACA intended to improve LTC financing, service delivery, and regulation. Here, I review the basic problems plaguing the LTC sector and the provisions promulgated within the ACA to address them. I conclude with a brief overview of the issue's content.

THE LTC DILEMMA

LTC in the United States is hampered by several challenges. Problematic areas include a lack of financial preparation and ability to pay for the high costs of services. They also include inadequate care coordination, which compromises care quality and costs, particularly among the Medicare-Medicaid dually eligible. There has also been insufficient progress toward rebalancing LTC toward greater use of noninstitutional alternatives to nursing home placement. Recruitment and retention of a well-trained, stable workforce remains problematic as well; so too does the continuing provision of poor quality care by a large proportion of providers.

Financing and Insurance

Two-thirds of specialists surveyed as part of the Commonwealth Fund LTC Opinion Leader Survey ranked "financing" among the top three challenges facing LTC (Miller et al., 2010). In 2011, the average annual cost of institutional LTC ranged from $41,724 for assisted living to $78,110 for a semiprivate room in a nursing home and $83,585 for a private room (Mature Market Institute, 2011). The average annual cost of community-based care included $18,200 for 5 days of adult day services and $27,664 to $30,576 for 4 hours of homemaker, companion, and/or home health services, 7 days per week. Relatively few have given much, if any, thought about how to pay for LTC needs that arise during retirement (Kaiser Family Foundation, 2007). Consequently, comparatively few have purchased private insurance or accumulated enough assets to assist with those expenses should they arise. Only 10% of elderly people and 7 million non-elderly adults have a private LTC insurance policy (Melnyk, 2005). Only one-third of elderly people have sufficient levels of assets to pay for 1 year of nursing home care (Lyons, Schneider, & Desmond, 2005). Since 27% of current workers report less than $1,000 in savings and investments and 54% have less than $25,000, it is likely that future generations of retirees will lack sufficient resources to pay for the expenses associated with LTC as well (Helman, Copeland, & VanDerhei, 2010).

Overall, 29% of the nation's $264 billion in LTC costs were paid out-of-pocket in 2008 and just 7% through private insurance (Shugarman & Steenhausen, 2010). Furthermore, the majority of formal LTC expenses were paid for by government, either through Medicaid (40%) or Medicare (20%). Both programs are limited, however. Medicare pays for post-acute and rehabilitation services only. While Medicaid serves as a safety net for those requiring care over longer periods of time, it requires potential recipients to impoverish themselves, or accrue medical expenses in excess of their income, before they can qualify for program benefits. Furthermore, requirements for Medicaid eligibility vary substantially from state to state, with respect to both the financial and functional eligibility criteria applied. Due in part to limited ability to pay for formal services and supports, most Americans with LTC needs receive unpaid, informal care only (Kaye et al., 2010). This was valued at $450 billion in 2009 (Feinberg, Reinhard, Houser, & Choula, 2011).

HCBS

Most frail and chronically ill older adults would prefer to remain at home as long as possible. This is also the preference of the broader policy community, with, for example, 84% of LTC specialists—consumer advocates, providers, policy experts, government officials—believing that the LTC system should be rebalanced away from institutions toward HCBS (Miller et al., 2010). Currently, there are nearly 2 million elderly individuals in the community in need of care on par with that required by the nation's 1.8 million nursing home residents (Cigolle, Langa, Kabeto, & Blaum, 2005). Due to a lack of available services and supports, however, a large proportion of prevailing need goes unmet, including one in five community-dwelling adults with limitations in activities of dialing living (Komisar, Feder, & Kasper, 2005). Moreover, between 5.1% and 11.8% of long-stay nursing home residents and 5.2% and 13.5% of new admissions can be categorized as low-care, suggesting that a non-negligible proportion could be transferred back to the community, or prevented from going in to a nursing home in the first place, if sufficient services and supports were made available (Mor et al., 2007).

That LTC rebalancing has become a policy priority is reflected in the Supreme Court's 1999 decision in *Olmstead v. LC* and a number of federal and state initiatives, not least of which include Medicaid HCBS waivers, consumer direction, and the Money Follows the Person Demonstration (Miller, Allen, & Mor, 2009; Shirk, 2006). The result has been considerable growth, with Medicaid HCBS program participants and expenditures increasing from 1.9 to 2.8 million and $17 to $42 billion, respectively, between 1999 and 2007 (Ng & Harrington, 2011). Yet despite such progress there is still a long way to go. Currently, for example, there are more than 365,000 people on waitlists for HCBS waivers in 39 states (Ng & Harrington, 2011). Moreover, just 33.8% of Medicaid LTC spending for aged and disabled individuals is devoted to home- and community-based care (Eiken, Sredl, Burwell, & Gold, 2010). Most Medicaid LTC spending is still directed toward nursing homes.

Workforce Instability

Recruitment and retention of a well-trained, stable workforce is critical for ensuring the provision of sufficient levels of high-quality LTC as the population ages. Indeed, "workforce" was ranked as the most pressing challenge facing LTC by specialists working in this area (Miller et al., 2010). Perhaps the prominence assigned to workers derives from a larger body of research demonstrating a relationship between the type and quantity of staffing and quality of care received (Bostick, Rantz, Flesner, & Riggs, 2006; Centers for Medicare and Medicaid Services [CMS], 2002; Stone, 2004). But despite its importance, staff turnover rates in home care range from 40% to 60% and in nursing homes, it is two-thirds or more for some staff categories (American Health Care Association, 2008; PHI, 2005). There is also a growing gap in "care capacity." More than 422,000 additional nurse aides, orderlies, and attendants; 552,000 home health aides; and 477,000 personal and home care aides will be needed over the next 10 years (U.S. Bureau of Labor Statistics, 2010).

Challenges recruiting and retaining direct care staff derive from a number of factors, including poor public perception, the demanding nature of the work, perceived lack of value and respect, insufficient training and autonomy, and limited opportunities for career advancement (CMS, 2002; Mickus, Luz, & Hogan, 2004; Miller & Mor, 2007). The LTC workforce is also among the most poorly compensated in the nation. With a median hourly wage of $10.58 in 2009, direct care workers earned substantially less than other U.S. workers ($15.95) (PHI, 2011). They are also more than two times as likely as other workers to be low-income or live in poverty (68.0% vs. 30.0%; Smith & Baughman, 2007). Moreover, few direct care workers have access to health insurance coverage, vacation time, tuition assistance, child care, pensions, and other benefits (Fishman, Barnow, Glosser, & Gardiner, 2004; Smith & Baughman, 2007). In 2011, for example, 900,000 direct care workers lacked health insurance coverage, including one-quarter working in nursing homes and one-third working in agency-based home care (PHI, 2011).

Quality Assurance and Improvement

For many, insufficient quality is the crux of what is wrong with the nation's LTC system. Although progress has been made in improving federal and state oversight and levels of quality in the 2 decades following the passage of nursing home quality reform with the Omnibus Budget Reconciliation Act of 1987, substantial challenges remain (Castle & Ferguson, 2010; Wiener et al., 2007). In 2010, for example, 93.9% of nursing facilities received at least one deficiency citation, while one-quarter (23.4%) received one or more citations for deficiencies that resulted in actual harm or immediate jeopardy for residents (Harrington, Carrillo, Dowdell, Tang, & Blank, 2011). The Administration on Aging's Ombudsmen Program investigated 211,937 complaints from nursing home, board and care home, and assisted living facility residents and other individuals that year (Administration on Aging, 2011).

Especially problematic is considerable interstate variation in the number and severity of deficiencies and the application of civil monetary penalties and other sanctions despite the existence of federal standards (Harrington, Mullan, & Carrillo, 2004; Miller & Mor, 2008). Continuing uncertainty about the use of nursing home quality indicators also exists, with regard to both breadth, validity, and reliability and to their use in public reporting and pay-for-performance (Castle & Ferguson, 2010; Mor, 2005). These challenges are especially salient today as nursing home residents are increasingly frail and debilitated and medically more complex (Decker, 2005; National Nursing Home Survey, 2010). Similar issues extend to assisted living and home- and community-based providers, particularly since they have been subject to far less scrutiny than nursing homes. Ongoing concern about the quality of LTC and efforts to assure and improve it is reflected in polls, both of the general public and of specialists who work in this area professionally (Kaiser Family Foundation, 2007; Miller et al., 2010).

Chronic Care Coordination and the Dually Eligible

About 91% of those aged 65 years and older in 2006 had at least one chronic health condition; nearly three-quarters had two or more (Anderson, 2010). The presence of multiple chronic conditions increases the risk of disability and physical impairment. It is also associated with increased prescription drug use, physician contacts, home health visits, and hospitalizations. The result is increased health care expenditures, with nearly all Medicare spending, for example—79%—deriving from care provided to beneficiaries with five or more conditions (Anderson, 2010). Those with chronic illnesses frequently experience difficulty coordinating care across multiple providers.

They also frequently experience inadequate transitions across care settings. Together, lack of coordination and poor transitions increase the likelihood of duplication, fragmentation, lack of care continuity, care delays, medication errors, and other adverse events (Coleman, Smith, Raha, & Min, 2005; Schoen et al., 2011). Largely because of gaps in care that occur as a result of missing information, many patients transferred from hospitals to nursing homes or paid home care are quickly rehospitalized (Coleman, 2003; Murtaugh & Litke, 2002). This is particularly true of those with chronic conditions, with the number of potentially avoidable hospitalizations increasing from 1 per 1,000 Medicare beneficiaries 65 years and older with one chronic condition to 66 per 1,000 for those with five chronic conditions and 530 per 1,000 for those with 10 or more (Anderson, 2010). In all, approximately 20% of Medicare patients, or 2.6 million seniors, discharged from hospitals are readmitted within 30 days at a cost in excess of $26 billion per year (HealthCare.gov, 2011).

Concerns about care coordination are further exacerbated among the 8.9 million individuals dually eligible for Medicare and Medicaid (Kaiser Family Foundation, 2011). Dually eligible individuals are substantially more likely than other Medicare beneficiaries to be low-income, in fair or poor health, cognitively/mentally impaired, impaired in activities of daily living, and chronically ill (Anderson, 2010; Kasper, Watts, & Lyons, 2010). They are also substantially more likely to use health care services of varying types. Thus, while the dually eligible constitute 15% of Medicaid enrollment, they represent 39% of total Medicaid spending (Kaiser Family Foundation, 2011). Being dually eligible also exacerbates the spending impact of chronic illness: Medicare spends substantially more for those who are dually eligible than for Medicare-only beneficiaries with similar numbers of chronic conditions (Kasper et al., 2010). In 2008, for example, dually eligible beneficiaries with five or more chronic conditions had considerably higher per capita Medicare spending ($54,199) than other Medicare beneficiaries with five or more conditions ($38,675; The SCAN Foundation, 2010). Especially concerning is the prevailing lack of coordination between Medicare and Medicaid, particularly with respect to the provision of acute and long-term services to dual beneficiaries (Grabowski, 2007; Miller & Wiessert, 2003). Conflicting incentives that inhibit coordination between these and other programs need to be addressed.

THE AFFORDABLE CARE ACT AND LTC

The most prominent LTC-related provision in the ACA is the now-suspended CLASS Act. Other pertinent provisions include additional incentives and options for expanding Medicaid HCBS, a number of research and demonstration projects, particularly in the areas of chronic care coordination and the dually eligible, and a grab bag of nursing home quality reforms. There are also provisions that could improve the quality of the LTC workforce. Benefit improvements and spending reductions under Medicare were included as well.

Prioritizing LTC Financing: The CLASS Act

If implementation of the CLASS Act had not been abandoned by the Obama Administration, it would have resulted in the creation of government-run LTC insurance program. The ACA established the general parameters of the program including, in relation to CLASS enrollment, premiums, benefit triggers, coverage levels, and administration. In short, the CLASS program would have been open to everyone aged 18 years or older who worked and met minimal earnings requirements. No underwriting would have been allowed; premiums would have varied solely on the basis of age, although the working poor and certain full-time students would have been required to make nominal contributions. Individuals could have enrolled in the CLASS plan either individually or through their employers. Should their employers have participated, workers would have automatically been enrolled unless they opted out. To qualify for CLASS benefits, enrollees would have had to have contributed 5 years' worth of premiums, during 3 of which they would have been required to earn enough income to be credited for one-quarter of Social Security benefits ($1,120 in 2011). To receive CLASS benefits, an individual would have had to have had at least two or three impairments in activities of daily living, cognitive impairment, or their equivalent. CLASS enrollees would have received a minimum average cash benefit of $50 per day, scaled to level of functional ability and indexed to inflation. The ACA limited costs associated with administering CLASS to no more than 3% of all premiums paid. It also explicitly excluded the federal treasury as a potential revenue source. Premiums could have been adjusted upward to maintain the fiscal soundness of the program.

Encouraging Progress Toward LTC Rebalancing

The ACA addresses Medicaid's continuing institutional bias by incentivizing and extending a number of Medicaid HCBS options in addition to addressing such issues as spousal impoverishment, information dissemination, and nursing home transitions. The ACA extends mandatory spousal impoverishment protections to community-based spouses of people receiving HCBS. It authorizes additional funds for Aging Disability and Resource Centers that provide single points of entry into LTC. It extends the Money Follows the Person Demonstration and shortens the requirement for residency in a nursing home from 6 months to 90 days for residents to qualify. Most importantly, perhaps, there are additional incentives and options for states to expand HCBS options under Medicaid, including the State Balancing Incentive Payments program, which provides for enhanced federal matching payments from 2011 to 2015 for states increasing the proportion of spending on HCBS; a new Medicaid state plan option for attendant services and supports known as the Community First Choice Option; and modifications to the little-used 1915(i) state plan option first promulgated under the Deficit Reduction Act of 2005.

Enhancing Workforce Recruitment and Retention

The ACA includes provisions affecting both professional and paraprofessional workers in a variety of settings, including nursing homes, personal attendants, and family care. There are also a number of demonstration projects and grants in this area, not to mention the expansion of health insurance coverage to previously uninsured direct care staff. Specific provisions include enhanced training for certified nurse assistants on dementia and abuse in nursing homes and a national program on criminal background checks for LTC workers in a variety of settings. Provisions meant to enhance the personal care workforce were included in the CLASS Act, which would have allowed beneficiaries to pay family caregivers and required states to assess the existing infrastructure in this area. Specific demonstrations and grants include a six-state demonstration to develop core competencies, pilot curricula, and certification programs for personal and home care aides, in addition to grants for career ladder programs for nurses, nurse assistants, and home health aides. Money is allocated for geriatric education centers to support training for faculty in health professional schools, direct care workers, and family caregivers. Importantly, the ACA will provide most direct care workers with health insurance coverage through the combination of the individual mandate, Medicaid expansion, low-income subsidies, employer penalties, and insurance exchanges.

Improving Nursing Home Quality

The ACA includes a number of provisions meant to increase transparency in the nursing home sector, in addition to several demonstration projects and other initiatives with which to better ensure and improve quality and prevent elder abuse and neglect. Transparency is increased through disclosure of more detailed information about ownership, staffing, and expenditures, implementation of compliance and ethics programs, improvements to the Nursing Home Compare website, and adoption of a standardized complaint form. Other nursing home–related provisions are national demonstrations on culture change and the use of information technology in nursing homes. There are provisions that promote pay-for-performance as well. Although the demonstration of pay-for-performance in Medicare is in progress, the

ACA requires the U.S. Department of Health and Human Services to develop an implementation plan for adopting this approach in the Medicare skilled nursing facility program more generally. Provisions meant to improve the quality and training of direct care workers, a component of nursing home quality, were already discussed.

Enhancing Care for the Dually Eligible and Other Medicare Beneficiaries

To improve chronic care coordination, the ACA establishes new offices within the CMS. It also reauthorizes Medicare Special Needs Plans (SNPs) while authorizing a number of pertinent research and demonstration projects. Relevant administrative changes include the establishment of the Federal Coordinated Health Care Office and the Center for Medicare and Medicaid Innovation within CMS, with the former being charged with improving coordination between Medicare and Medicaid and the latter with testing innovative payment and delivery arrangements with successful models being permitted to be implemented nationally without additional legislation. The ACA also reauthorized SNPs, which are Medicare advantage plans that target enrollment of beneficiaries who are dually eligible, nursing home residents, or those with chronically disabling conditions. From now on SNPs must contract with both Medicare and Medicaid. Pertinent demonstrations addressing chronic care coordination for the broader Medicare population are included in the ACA too. These encompass medical homes, payment bundling, and end-of-life care.

Other provisions that may enhance care for Medicare beneficiaries more generally include closing the gap in Part D prescription drug coverage (i.e., the "donut hole"), improving coverage for preventive care and wellness visits, and increasing payments to primary care physicians. On the other hand, the ACA reduces payments to private plans under Medicare Advantage, which have been overpaid relative to traditional fee-for-service Medicare (Biles, Pozen, & Gutterman, 2009). It also provides a significant source of funding for health care reform by slowing down the rate of growth in payments for many non-physician Medicare program benefits, including outpatient hospital, skilled nursing facility, home health, and hospice care. A 15-member independent payment advisory board was established to recommend areas for cost savings as well. Additional revenues will be generated through the establishment and increase in income-related premiums under Medicare Parts B and D, respectively.

ISSUE CONTENT

This issue includes three articles on the CLASS Act and its implications by Joshua M. Wiener, William G. Weissert, and Mark Meiners. It also includes an article on the ACA's HCBS provisions by Charlene Harrington and colleagues, potential enhancements to the LTC workforce by Robyn Stone and Natasha Bryant, improvements to the quality of nursing home care by Catherine Hawes and associates, care coordination for the dually eligible by David Grabowski, and broader Medicare program changes by Marilyn Moon.

Wiener believes that fate of the CLASS Act provides useful lessons for future efforts to reform LTC financing. Although implementation has been suspended, the debate over CLASS highlights choices the government must make with any public LTC insurance program. This includes, with respect to preventing adverse selection, setting premiums, determining eligibility, triggering benefits, establishing benefit levels, undertaking marketing, and addressing the relationship with private LTC insurance. Decisions regarding elements such as these will largely determine whether the general working population can be educated to recognize the risk of needing LTC as they age, whether they believe a program such as CLASS can help to meet future LTC needs—that is, a program that offers value for its cost—and whether the working population can afford the premiums. The experience with CLASS also raises the issue of whether there should be one age-blind LTC insurance system or whether younger disabled people should be considered separately from older adults.

Weissert argues that the CLASS Act gave the impression that it would finance baby boomers' nursing home care needs—a financial burden overwhelming families and bankrupting the states. But the CLASS Act was designed to pay for HCBS. Its average $50-a-day cash payment would not have been nearly enough to cover the $6,000- to $7,000-a-month cost of nursing home care. Few people have saved enough to pay for these costs; consequently, most must rely on Medicaid after spending down their income and assets. Furthermore, CLASS assumed that HCBS could be used to ward off nursing home entry despite decades of research demonstrating little to no substitution effect. Now that experience with CLASS has shown just how difficult it is to deal with the selection and financing challenges associated with LTC, it is unlikely that Congress will revisit the issue in the foreseeable future to address the true catastrophic risk of LTC, namely, nursing home placement.

Meiners believes that useful lessons can be drawn from the private LTC insurance market and State Partnership Programs, which incentivize LTC insurance purchases through the provision of more generous Medicaid eligibility requirements, about how to make CLASS fiscally viable. CLASS's "long and lean" benefit structure would have provided a small daily cash benefit for as long as someone needed LTC. Providing potential enrollees with a single option such as this is unlikely to draw in as many subscribers as possible. Doing so requires offering multiple plan options that appeal to different segments of market risk. Thus, CLASS might draw in more enrollees by making additional options available to the basic CLASS plan, including one that appealed to those who preferred catastrophic protection and one that appealed to those desiring a more generous benefit over a limited period of time. Revising CLASS in this way could have enlarged the risk pool, reduced adverse selection, and lowered program costs.

Harrington, Ng, LaPlante, and Kaye observe that the Community First Choice Option, revised 1915(i) state plan benefit, and State Balancing Incentive Payments program provide important, voluntary options and incentives for Medicaid HCBS expansion. However, the impact of these initiatives will likely be limited. While some states have made substantial progress toward rebalancing, others have not, particularly for the aged and disabled. Since the law does not set minimum standards for access to HCBS benefits or require states to cover all target groups, unmet need among certain populations will continue. Moreover, some states may be unwilling to make the structural changes necessary to administer HCBS and to accept additional federal reporting requirements. The new incentives also may not be sufficient to encourage major changes in light of ongoing state budget difficulties. Wide variations in access to HCBS can be expected to continue while such care competes with mandated institutional care for funding.

Stone and Bryant point out that the ACA is the first major piece of federal legislation to recognize the need to increase the number of geriatrically trained health professionals and direct care workers. However, the legislation is limited in its ability to generate the supply necessary to meet the caregiving demands associated with population aging and the new service delivery models instituted by the ACA. Currently, the professional workforce lacks the requisite skills, knowledge, competencies, and training necessary to coordinate and integrate care in the manner suggested by the new models specified in the legislation. The ACA also neglects to address some of the major barriers to recruiting and retaining direct care workers, including non-competitive compensation and benefits (with the exception of basic health insurance coverage) and an unsatisfactory work environment. Furthermore, several of the pertinent provisions have not received appropriations. Most are also demonstration projects of limited scope and duration.

Hawes and colleagues identify a number of elements within the ACA that could affect the quality of care delivered in nursing homes. The aim is to improve quality and reduce abuse and neglect of residents by increasing the transparency of information, enhancing facility accountability and capacity, improving the quality and skills of staff, and strengthening quality assurance mechanisms. Most of these provisions were originally parts of bills—the Elder Justice Act and the Nursing Home Transparency and Improvement Act—introduced in multiple sessions of Congress but that never garnered sufficient attention or support to pass on their own, particularly in light of ongoing industry opposition. It was not until these bills were folded into the broader health reform effort that they were passed into law. The legislative history of these two acts suggests that the political vulnerability of nursing home reform remains as implementation begins to unfold, in terms of overcoming industry opposition, insufficient congressional appropriations, and a lack of urgency on the part of certain implementing agencies.

Grabowski highlights demonstrations being developed by the Federal Coordinated Health Care Office and Center for Medicare and Medicaid Innovation to promote integrated care for dually eligible beneficiaries. Foremost among these is the State Demonstrations to Integrate Care for Dual Eligibles Program, through which 15 states have been awarded federal funding to develop better ways to coordinate care for the dually eligible. Because a wide range of payment and service delivery model reforms have been proposed by participating states, the demonstration should provide an excellent opportunity with which to identify the most cost-effective approaches for integrating care for this population. Four principles that might influence the success of these and other nascent initiatives to coordinate care include pairing delivery and payment reforms, being sure to engage Medicaid as well as Medicare, considering shifting responsibility for the dually eligible entirely onto Medicare or Medicaid, and mandating compulsory enrollment in managed care.

Moon focuses on non–LTC-related changes made by the ACA that affect senior and disabled Medicare beneficiaries. She points out that the ACA made modest benefit improvements to Medicare while largely underwriting health care reform by restraining the rate of growth in Medicare spending over time. Although the expansions in benefits enacted in such areas as prescriptions drugs, preventive care, and wellness are important, the ACA still leaves the Medicare program with a less comprehensive benefit package than many receive through their employer-sponsored health insurance policies. Moon argues that the negative consequences of spending reductions on Medicare providers and beneficiaries is overstated, that greater proportional reductions were made in the past, and that the same reductions would likely have been considered as part of deficit reduction anyway. The changes made should extend the life of the Part A trust fund, thereby placing the program on stronger financial footing.

CONCLUSION

In incorporating LTC into the ACA, it was the sense of the Senate that "Congress should address long-term services and supports in a comprehensive way that guarantees elderly and disabled individuals the care they need" (Title II, Subtitle E, Section 2406). But just how effective is the ACA likely to be in addressing the challenges facing LTC? Will it result in meaningful reform or will it just tinker around the edges? This special issue of *Journal of Aging & Social Policy* seeks to answer these questions by drawing on the knowledge and insights of our expert contributors. The general view is that the CLASS Act provides useful lessons for LTC financing reform, although its implementation has been put on hold, likely permanently. Furthermore, while the ACA generally makes marginal changes in the other areas highlighted—HCBS, workforce, quality, dual eligibility, and Medicare—it reflects some progress toward addressing the problems underlying LTC provision in the United States, perhaps laying the ground work for further, more comprehensive reform in future years.

REFERENCES

Administration on Aging. (2011). *Long-term care ombudsman program.* Washington, DC: Author. Retrieved from www.aoa.gov/AoAroot/Press_Room/ Products_Materials/fact/ pdf/LTC_Ombudsman_Program_2011.pdf.

American Health Care Association. (2008). *Report of findings 2007 AHCA survey nursing staff and vacancy and turnover in nursing facilities.* Washington, DC: Author. Retrieved from www.ahcancal.org/research_data/staffing/documents/ vacancy_turnover_survey2007.pdf.

Anderson, G. (2010). *Chronic care: Making the case for ongoing care.* Princeton, NJ: Robert Wood Johnson Foundation. Retrieved from www.rwjf.org/files/research/ 50968chronic.care.chartbook.pdf.

Biles, B., Pozen, J., & Gutterman, S. (2009). *The continuing cost of privitization: Extra payments to Medicare Advantage plans jump to $11.4 billion in 2009.* New York, NY: The Commonwealth Fund. Retrieved from http://www. commonwealthfund.org/~/media/Files/Publications/Issue%20Brief/2009/May/ 1265_Biles_Extra_Payments_54_v2.pdf.

Bostick, J. E., Rantz, M., Flesner, K., & Riggs, C. J. (2006). Systematic review of studies of staffing and quality in nursing homes. *Journal of the American Medical Directors Association, 7*(6), 366–376.

Castle, N. G., & Ferguson, J. C. (2010). What is nursing home quality and how is it measured? *The Gerontologist, 50*(4), 426–442.

Centers for Medicare and Medicaid Services. (2002). *Appropriateness of minimum nurse staffing ratios in nursing homes phase ii final report.* Baltimore, MD: CMS.

Cigolle, C. T., Langa, K. M., Kabeto, M. U., & Blaum, C. S. (2005). Setting eligibility criteria for a care-coordination benefit. *Journal of the American Geriatrics Society, 53*(12), 2051–2059.

Coleman, E. A. (2003). Falling through the cracks: Challenges and opportunities for improving transitional care for persons with continuous complex care needs. *Journal of the American Geriatrics Society, 51*(4), 549–555.

Coleman, E. A., Smith, J. D., Raha, D., & Min, S. J. (2005). Posthospital medication discrepancies: Prevalence and contributing factors. *Archives of Internal Medicine, 165*(16), 1842–1847.

Decker, F. (2005). *Nursing homes, 1977–99: What has changed, what has not?* Hyattsville, MD: National Center for Health Statistics. Retrieved from www.cdc. gov/NCHS/data/nnhsd/NursingHomes1977_99.pdf.

Eiken, S., Sredl, K., Burwell, B., & Gold, L. (2010). *Medicaid long-term care expenditures in FY 2009*. Cambridge, MA: Thomas Healthcare. Retrieved from www.hcbs.org/moreInfo.php/doc/3325.

Federal Interagency Forum on Aging Related Statistics. (2010). *Older Americans 2010: Key indicators of well-being*. Retrieved from www.agingstats.gov/Main_Site/Data/2010_Documents/docs/Introduction.pdf.

Feinberg, L., Reinhard, S. C., Houser, A., & Choula, R. (2011). *Valuing the invaluable: 2011 update, the growing contributions of family caregiving*. Washington, DC. AARP Public Policy Institute. Retrieved from http://assets.aarp.org/rgcenter/ppi/ltc/i51-caregiving.pdf.

Fishman, M. F., Barnow, B., Glosser, A., & Gardiner, K. (2004). *Recruiting and retaining a quality paraprofessional long-term care workforce*. Washington, DC: U.S. Department of Health and Human Services. Retrieved from http://aspe.hhs.gov/daltcp/reports/natwis.pdf.

Gleckman, H. (2011). Requiem for the CLASS Act. *Health Affairs, 30*(12), 2231–2234.

Grabowski, D. C. (2007). Medicare and Medicaid: Conflicting incentives for long-term care. *The Milbank Quarterly, 85*(4), 579–610.

Harrington, C., Carrillo, H., Dowdell, M., Tang, P. P., & Blank, B. W. (2011). *Nursing facility staffing, residents and facility deficiencies, 2005 through 2010*. Retrieved from www.aanhr.org/OSCAR%202011%20final.pdf.

Harrington, C., Mullan, J. T., & Carrillo, H. (2004). State nursing home enforcement systems. *Journal of Health Politics, Policy, & Law, 29*(1), 43–73.

HealthCare.gov. (2011). *Partnership for patients: Better care, lower costs*. Retrieved from www.healthcare.gov/news/factsheets/2011/04/partnership04122011a.html.

Helman, R., Copeland C., &VanDerhei, J. (2010). *The 2010 Retirement Confidence Survey: Confidence stabilizing, but preparations continue to erode*. Washington, DC. Employee Benefit Research Institute. Retrieved from www.ebri.org/surveys/rcs/2010/.

Kaiser Family Foundation. (2007). *Kaiser Public opinion spotlight: The public's views on long-term care*. Washington, DC: The Henry J. Kaiser Family Foundation. Retrieved from www.kff.org/kaiserpolls/upload/7719.pdf.

Kaiser Family Foundation. (2011, May). *Dual eligibles: Medicaid's role for low income Medicare beneficiaries*. Washington, DC: The Henry J. Kaiser Family Foundation. Retrieved from http://www.kff.org/medicaid/upload/4091-08.pdf.

Kasper, J., Watts, M. O., & Lyons, B. (2010). *Chronic disease and co-morbidity among dual eligibles: Implications for patterns of Medicaid and Medicare service use and spending*. Washington, DC: Kaiser Family Foundation. Retrieved from www.kff.org/medicaid/upload/8081.pdf.

Kaye, H. S., Harrington, C., & LaPlante, M. P. (2010). Long-term care: Who gets it, who provides it, who pays, and how much? *Health Affairs, 29*(1), 11–21.

Komisar, H. L., Feder J., & Kasper J. D. (2005). Unmet long-term care needs: An analysis of Medicare-Medicaid dual eligibles. *Inquiry, 42*(2), 171–182.

Lyons, B., Schneider, A., & Desmond, K. A. (2005). *The distributions of assets in he elderly population living in the community*. Retrieved from www.kff.org/medicaid/7335.cfm.

Mature Market Institute. (2011). *The 2011 MetLife market survey of nursing home, assisted living, adult day services, and home care costs*. Westport, CT: Author.

Retrieved from www.metlife.com/assets/cao/mmi/publications/studies/2011/
mmi-market-survey-nursing-home-assisted-living-adult-day-services-costs.pdf.

Melnyk, A. (2005). *Long-term care insurance or Medicaid: Who will pay for
baby boomers' long-term care?* Retrieved from www.acli.com/NR/rdonlyres/
FEB87D8A-9E2F-45B6-B08A-CBED882A66C6/0/LTCBabyBoomers05.pdf.

Mickus, M., Luz, C. C., & Hogan, A. (2004). *Voices from the front: Recruitment and
retention of direct care workers in long-term care across Michigan.* Lansing,
MI: Michigan State University. Retrieved from www.directcareclearinghouse.
org/download/MI_vocices_from_the_front.pdf.

Miller, E. A. (2011). flying beneath the radar of health reform: The Community
Living Assistance Services and Supports (CLASS) Act. *The Gerontologist, 51*(2),
145–155.

Miller, E. A., Allen, S. M., & Mor, V. (2009). Navigating the labyrinth of long-term
care: Shoring up informal caregiving in a home- and community-based world.
Journal of Aging & Social Policy, 21(1), 1–16.

Miller, E. A., & Mor, V. (2007). Trends and challenges in building a 21st century
long-term care workforce. In C. M. Mara (Ed.), *Handbook of long-term care
administration and policy* (pp. 133–156). Taylor & Francis CRC Press.

Miller, E. A., & Mor, V. (2008). Balancing regulatory controls and incentives: Toward
smarter and more transparent oversight in long-term care. *Journal of Health
Politics, Policy, and Law, 33*(2), 249–279.

Miller, E. A., Mor, V., & Clark, M. (2010). Reforming long-term care in the United
States: Findings from a national survey of specialists. *The Gerontologist, 50*(2),
238–252.

Miller, E. A., & Weissert, W. G. (2003). Strategies for Integrating Medicare and
Medicaid: Design Features and Incentives. *Medical Care Research & Review,
60*(2), 123–157.

Mor, V. (2005). Improving the quality of long-term care with better information. *The
Milbank Quarterly, 83*(3), 333–364.

Mor, V., Zinn, J., Gozalo, P, Feng, Z., Intrator, O., & Grabowski, D. C. (2007).
Prospects for transferring nursing home residents to the community. *Health
Affairs, 26*(6), 1762–1771.

Murtaugh, C. M., & Litke, A. (2002). Transitions through post-acute and long-term
care settings: Patterns of use and outcomes for a national cohort of elders.
Medical Care, 40(3), 227–236.

National Nursing Home Survey. (2010). *Trends in nursing home beds by size.*
Retrieved from www.cdc.gov/nchs/nnhs/nursing_home_trends.htm.

Ng, T., & Harrington, C. (2011). *Medicaid home- and community-based service programs: Data update.* Washington, DC: Kaiser Family Foundation. Retrieved from
www.kff.org/medicaid/upload/7720-04.pdf.

PHI. (2005). *The role of training in improving the recruitment and retention of
direct-care workers in long-term care.* Bronx, NY: PHI. Retrieved from www.
directcareclearinghouse.org/download/WorkforceStrategies3.pdf.

PHI. (2011). *Who are direct care workers?* Retrieved from www.
directcareclearinghouse.org/download/NCDCW%20Fact%20Sheet-1.pdf.

Schoen, C., Osborn, R., Squires, D., Doty, M. M., Pierson, R., & Applebaum, S.
(2011). New 2011 survey of patients with complex care needs in eleven

countries finds that care is often poorly coordinated. *Health Affairs, 30*(12), 2437–2448.

Shirk, C. (2006). *Rebalancing long-term care: The role of the Medicaid HCBS Waiver Program*. Retrieved from www.nhpf.org/library/background-papers/BP_HCBS. Waivers_03-03-06.pdf.

Shugarman, L. R., & Steenhausen, S. (2010). *The financing of long-term care*. Long Beach, CA: The SCAN Foundation.

Smith, K., & Baughman, R. (2007). Caring for America's aging population: A profile of the direct-care workforce. *Monthly Labor Review* (September), 20–26.

Stone, R. I. (2004). The direct care workers: The third rail of home care policy. *Annual Review of Public Health, 25*, 521–537.

The SCAN Foundation. (2010). *Dual eligibles and Medicare spending*. DataBrief Series, No. 3. Retrieved from www.thescanfoundation.org/sites/default/files/ 1pg_DataBrief_No3.pdf.

U.S. Bureau of Labor Statistics. (2010). *Selected occupational projections data*. Retrieved from http://data.bls.gov:8080/oep/servlet/oep.noeted.servlet. ActionServlet?Action=empeduc.

Wiener, J. M., Freiman, M. P., & Brown, D. (2007). *Nursing home care quality: twenty years after the Omnibus Budget Reconciliation Act of 1987*. Washington, DC: RTI. Retrieved from www.kff.org/medicare/upload/7717.pdf.

The CLASS Act: Is It Dead or Just Sleeping?

JOSHUA M. WIENER, PhD

*Distinguished Fellow and Program Director for Aging, Disability, and
Long-Term Care, RTI International, Washington, District of Columbia, USA*

*The Affordable Care Act (ACA) established a voluntary public
insurance program for long-term care: the Community Living
Assistance Services and Supports (CLASS) Act. In October 2011, the
Obama Administration announced that the program would not be
implemented because of the high risk of fiscal insolvency. Under the
legislative design, adverse selection was a major risk and premiums
would have been very high. This article discusses several CLASS Act
design and implementation issues, including the design features
that led to the decision not to implement the program: the voluntary enrollment, the weak work requirement, the lifetime and cash
benefits, and the premium subsidy for low-income workers and
students.*

INTRODUCTION

Title VIII of the Patient Protection and Affordable Care Act (ACA), the health
care reform legislation passed by Congress and signed by President Obama
in March 2010, established a voluntary public insurance program for long-
term care, the Community Living Assistance Services and Supports (CLASS)
Act. Championed by the late Senator Edward Kennedy, the CLASS program
was to be a "public option" for long-term care insurance. Although the CLASS

Act had the potential to radically change long-term care financing, it received little attention during the health care reform debate, and few people outside of a handful of long-term care experts knew about it (Miller, 2011).

On October 14, 2011, U.S. Department of Health and Human Services Secretary Kathleen Sebelius (2011) announced that the Obama Administration would not implement the CLASS Act program because it could not certify that the program would be actuarially sound and financially solvent for at least 75 years. At the heart of the problems were estimated premiums ranging from $235 to $391 per month, far too high to be affordable for the vast majority of working Americans (Greenlee, 2011). Although legal opinions varied on how much flexibility the secretary had to waive or modify statutory provisions, the magnitude of changes necessary to make the program financially solvent would have required very substantial deviation from the original statute (U.S. Department of Health and Human Services, 2011). Consumer advocates for older people and younger adults with disabilities are greatly disappointed, and opponents of health reform have cited the CLASS Act as emblematic of the overall problems of the ACA.

Although the CLASS Act will not be implemented in its original form, there is still much to be learned from its short life. After a brief description of the CLASS program to set the context, this paper analyzes the implementation problems that the program faced, particularly those that led to the decision not to start the program. Beyond these flaws, program administrators had to address several other difficult but not insurmountable issues, including how to enroll participants, how to link disability levels to payments, and whether restrictions should be placed on use of the cash benefit.

BACKGROUND

The CLASS Act drew heavily on the German and Japanese long-term care insurance programs (Campbell, Ikegami, & Gibson, 2010; Gibson & Redfoot, 2007). Table 1 summarizes the main elements of the CLASS Act insurance program as enacted. Most importantly, the program was voluntary; no one had to enroll if they did not want to. Except for full-time students, only working adults were eligible to participate. Unlike virtually all private long-term care insurance policies, the CLASS insurance program was not going to medically underwrite applicants. Thus, working people with disabilities and chronic medical illnesses would have been able to enroll. However, spousal and family coverage was not available, even with medical underwriting.

After paying premiums for at least 5 years, enrollees who met the disability threshold would have been eligible for a cash benefit, which would have averaged at least $50 a day, to help meet their long-term care needs. Benefits were to be provided on a lifetime basis without any limit on the benefit period or amount. The purpose of the 5-year waiting period was to

TABLE 1 Main Characteristics of the CLASS Act Insurance Program

The Community-Living Assistance Services and Supports (CLASS) Act insurance program is designed to provide insurance coverage for people with disabilities who need long-term care.

- The CLASS insurance program is a government insurance plan. It is the "public option" for long-term care.
- Initial enrollment is limited to people who are employed. Enrollment is on an individual basis and does not include spouses or children. Retirees who are not working are not eligible to enroll.
- Enrollment is voluntary. However, for people who work for participating employers, everyone will be automatically enrolled unless they choose not to participate. Other eligible adults will be enrolled on an individual basis via an alternative route.
- There is no medical underwriting for enrolling in the program, but enrollees must pay premiums for at least 5 years before they may receive benefits.
- To receive benefits, individuals must have a fairly severe level of disability. Enrollees must have at least two or three limitations in activities of daily living, cognitive impairment, or their equivalent. Determination of eligibility appears to rely heavily on documentation provided by physicians.
- Benefits vary by level of disability as determined by the secretary of the U.S. Department of Health and Human Services but will average no less than $50 per day and will be indexed to general inflation. Beneficiaries will have great flexibility in how they spend their benefit. Enrollees will be provided with assistance and counseling to navigate the program/service options. The benefit is not subject to any lifetime or aggregate limit.
- Insurance premiums are the sole source of financing. No general or earmarked taxes help to finance the program.
- The very low premiums for full-time students (ages 18 to 22) and people with incomes below the federal poverty level will be financed by subsidies by other insureds.
- No more than 3% of premiums may be used for administrative expenses. However, other funds may be used for administration of the program.
- Premiums will be set to maintain 75 years of program solvency.
- The CLASS program will supplement rather than replace other federal assistance. CLASS benefits will not count as income toward determining eligibility for other government programs. CLASS benefits will be the first payer for persons also eligible for Medicaid.

discourage people from waiting until they needed long-term care before they enrolled in the CLASS program. Moreover, individuals had to have worked at least 3 of the 5 years during this initial 5-year period. In addition, premiums had to continue to be paid after the 5-year waiting period to retain coverage, even if the person was not working. Failure to continue to pay premiums would have terminated the insurance coverage. Beneficiaries could have used the cash benefit to purchase supports and services, either from formal agencies or from individuals, including friends and family.

The insurance benefits were to be entirely financed by premiums; the program included no general government tax subsidy to lower the net cost of premiums as there is for Medicare Parts B or D. Students and working persons with incomes below the federal poverty level were scheduled to pay a monthly nominal premium of $5, but the cost of the subsidy would have been borne by other policy holders. Only 3% of premiums could be used for administrative costs, although there was no prohibition against using other appropriated government funds for this purpose. The law required the program to be fully self-financing over 75 years.

RATIONALE FOR THE CLASS ACT

Advocates for the CLASS Act noted that nursing home and extensive home care are very expensive; a year of nursing home care at private pay rates in 2010 cost an average of $67,525 per year, and home health agency aide care costs an average of $19 per hour (Genworth Financial, 2010). These expenses are beyond the financial reach of most Americans (Merlis, 2003; Wiener, Illston, & Hanley, 1994). Although Medicare covers short-term nursing home and home health care, it does not cover extended long-term care or services that do not require skilled nursing care. Although Medicaid serves as a safety net for those needing long-term care, program beneficiaries must meet stringent asset and income thresholds or incur large medical expenses before they can become eligible (Walker & Acciius, 2010). Despite an active market for almost 30 years, relatively few people have private long-term care insurance: only about 11% of people aged 55 and older in 2008 (Johnson & Park, 2011) and only about 2% of people aged 20 to 64 in 2005 (Feder, Komisar, & Friedland, 2007). As a result, long-term care is a major cause of catastrophic out-of-pocket cost, especially for older people.

The long-term care financing system is also biased toward institutional care, with 66% of 2009 Medicaid long-term care expenditures for older people and younger persons with physical disabilities being spent on nursing home care (Eiken, Kate, Burwell, & Gold, 2010). In addition, private long-term care insurance is medically underwritten, excluding people with disabilities and chronic illnesses, and has high levels of administrative costs relative to Medicare and Medicaid. If successful, CLASS would have brought additional revenues to the long-term care system, reduced dependence on Medicaid, and shifted services toward home- and community-based services.

While acknowledging the problems of the long-term care financing system, critics of the CLASS Act argued that a public program is unnecessary and undesirable or that design problems doomed the program to failure. Opponents contend that there is a viable private market for long-term care insurance and that public policy initiatives should focus on supporting it. Skeptics of the CLASS Act also questioned whether the voluntary nature of the CLASS Act insurance program, its lack of a broad government premium subsidy, and absence of medical underwriting would provide more affordable premiums than private-sector plans. As a result of these features, skeptics doubted whether the program could be financially stable over time. Finally, they noted that Medicare and Social Security face major financial problems, that health reform will require large new subsidies for health insurance, and that the federal government faces high levels of debt, reducing the desirability of starting a new program for which there is an implied federal financial guarantee.

DESIGN FEATURES THAT WOULD HAVE MADE CLASS INSOLVENT

Of particular importance to the program's demise were three broad factors: First, the lack of mandatory enrollment created problems of adverse selection that could not be resolved within the CLASS statutory framework. Second, the program contained features designed to address the needs of younger people with disabilities, but that did not fit a self-financed program. And third, the statute provided for extensive premium subsidies for the low-income population, but without the tax financing that normally goes with these types of subsidies. All three of these design features would have substantially increased premiums.

The Problem of Voluntary Programs

Unlike public long-term care insurance programs in countries such as Japan, Germany, and the Netherlands, the CLASS insurance program did not require that everyone participate. With the resistance to a mandate for general health insurance, it was probably inevitable that CLASS be a voluntary program. As a result, however, the program would have been potentially subject to adverse selection, which would have driven up the cost of premiums, possibly creating an insurance death spiral. Without medical underwriting to exclude them, people with disabilities who need long-term care and those at high risk for needing long-term care may have disproportionately enrolled in the program because the premiums would have been less than the out-of-pocket cost of the services that they believed they would use. To the extent that people without disabilities would not enroll because they did not believe that they had a substantial risk and that they would not receive important benefits, the program's ability to spread the costs of people using benefits across a broad population would have been limited. The resulting premiums would have been high, thereby causing people without disabilities not to enroll or to cancel enrollment, which would have further increased premiums and, in turn, caused more nondisabled people to cancel enrollment, further increasing premiums. The SCAN Foundation/Avalere Health long-term care insurance simulator estimates that the average premium for a mandatory long-term care insurance program with some features similar to the CLASS Act would be one-fourth of what it would be for a voluntary program, primarily because more people without disabilities would be enrolled (SCAN Foundation/Avalere Health, 2010).

To increase enrollment rates and reduce adverse selection, for employers who agreed to administer payroll deductions for CLASS insurance premiums, all workers would have been automatically enrolled. Individuals who did not want to enroll could opt out, but they had to explicitly decide to do so. This approach to increasing enrollment rates draws on behavioral economics research on participation in 401(k) retirement plans, which found that retirement savings enrollment rates are much higher when employees are required to opt out rather than opt in (Madrian & Shea, 2000).

The problem was that employers were not required to administer CLASS Act payroll deductions for employees. As a result, it was widely believed that the vast majority of employers would choose not to participate because they do not want the administrative burden, they are philosophically opposed to a public long-term care insurance program, or they already offer private long-term care insurance to their employees. Most importantly, employers may not have wanted to participate because automatic enrollment would be opposed by at least some employees, causing resentment toward the employer. Inducing employers to take on this administrative task would have been a difficult task, requiring an active marketing campaign to convince them that automatic enrollment was in their and their employees' best interest and that few employees would object. For those who work for organizations that choose not to offer payroll deductions and automatic enrollment, the program would have had to find ways to handle individual enrollment, perhaps through Social Security offices, mail, or websites.

Setting the CLASS program premiums was a classic "chicken and egg" problem. If actuaries assumed that large numbers of people would enroll and stay enrolled—including substantial numbers of people without long-term care needs or with a low likelihood of having such needs—then premiums would have been relatively low, and large numbers of people, including those without current or anticipated long-term care needs, would have likely enrolled. Advocates for the CLASS Act pointed to the near-universal enrollment in Medicare Part B (largely physician services) and Part D (prescription drugs) and the low prevalence of disability among workers as evidence that enrollment levels for the CLASS Act would have been high among nondisabled people.

Conversely, if actuaries assumed that relatively few people without current or anticipated long-term care needs would enroll and that most people with current or anticipated long-term care needs would have enrolled, then premiums would be high and few people without current or anticipated long-term care needs would participate. Those who argue this position noted that voluntary enrollment in private long-term care insurance policies in employment settings is low, with generally only about 5% to 7% of workers signing up. Premium estimates, primarily developed during the health care reform debate, assumed low levels of enrollment resulting in high average premiums ranging from $123 to $240 per month (American Academy of

Actuaries, 2009; Foster, 2010; Munnell & Hurwitz, 2011; U.S. Congressional Budget Office, 2010). The statute allows premiums to vary by age, and these previously estimated premiums have a fairly high average age. At younger ages, premiums would have been considerably below these averages.

A key problem for the CLASS Act program was that if premiums were $235 to $391 per month, as estimated by the Department of Health and Human Services (Greenlee, 2011), they would have been higher than premiums for private long-term care insurance for comparable benefits, albeit with medical underwriting (Tumlinson, Aguiar, & Watts, 2009). As a result, healthy workers might have preferred to purchase less expensive private insurance policies. The initial premium might well have created a self-fulfilling prophecy that could have determined the program's success or failure.

Meeting the Needs of Younger Adults With Disabilities

Because they do not work, the CLASS Act excluded retired older people and most younger adults with disabilities from participating in the program. The CLASS Act attempted to ease the sting of this design feature by establishing a weak work requirement that would let more people with disabilities enroll, providing lifetime benefits, and establishing a cash rather than service benefit. All of these features substantially increased the projected premiums.

First, the definition of "working" was too weak to prevent large numbers of people with disabilities from participating in the program. Because most people with disabilities are not in the workforce, it was expected that most would not have been able to enroll in CLASS. Under a broad definition of disability about 29% of people with disabilities work, accounting for only about 3% of the workforce (Kaye, 2010). Under a more restrictive definition, people with daily living and cognitive impairment disabilities accounted for 0.79% and 0.43% of the workforce, respectively. Retirees, people with disabilities not in the labor force, and nonworking spouses or partners could not participate, even with medical underwriting. This provision was meant to exclude most people who currently need long-term care services, reducing the amount of revenue needed to be raised to pay for services. Although many people in need of services who are not in the workforce initially would have been excluded from enrolling, the expectation was that over time, as enrollees age—and their risk for needing long-term care increases—the program would cover an increasing proportion of the population in need.

The problem was that the work requirement was very minimal, which meant that many people with disabilities could have qualified as working even if their attachment to the labor force was very tenuous. Individuals only had to earn enough to have one quarter credited for Social Security eligibility ($1,120 in 2011) during each of 3 years. Requiring higher levels of earnings would have excluded more younger adults with disabilities, reducing premiums. For example, in 2009, the median earnings of people without disabilities were $28,983, but only $18,865 for people with disabilities, about a third less (U.S. Census Bureau, 2010). People with intellectual disabilities and with severe mental illnesses, whose employment is often through sheltered workshops and who work relatively few hours, would probably have been the most affected if the earnings requirement were raised. While raising the work standard would probably lessen adverse selection, it would have also reduced the ability of CLASS to provide coverage to people who could not otherwise qualify for private long-term care insurance.

Second, like most government social programs, such as Medicaid and Social Security, CLASS was structured to provide benefits for as long as people needed them—in other words, lifetime benefits. Although lifetime coverage is particularly important to younger persons with disabilities who need coverage for the rest of their lives, lifetime coverage for private long-term care insurance is much more expensive than shorter periods of coverage. For example, for the Federal Long-Term Care Insurance Plan, lifetime coverage is more than a third more expensive than 5 years of coverage; it is more than twice the cost of 2 years of coverage (U.S. Office of Personnel Management, 2011). Private long-term care insurers typically offer policy holders the option of purchasing 1 year to lifetime coverage. However, only about 10% of policies purchased in 2009 provided lifetime benefits (American Association for Long-Term Care Insurance, 2010).

Third, and finally, to give program beneficiaries the greatest flexibility in obtaining services that met their individual needs, benefits were to be provided in cash rather than services. Although not limited to younger people with disabilities, the use of cash benefits and participant-directed care has been most aggressively advocated for that population (Wiener & Sullivan, 1995). Although there is an issue of how much accountability and what restrictions would have been required for the cash benefit (to be discussed below), actuaries typically assume that beneficiaries prefer cash to services and thus are more likely to claim the benefit. In other words, not everyone wants a stranger to come to their house to give them a bath, but almost everyone wants money, so the use of benefits is higher. In addition, in circumstances where providers have a shortage of workers, people authorized to receive service benefits may not actually be able to receive the benefits, as was the case in the Arkansas Cash and Counseling Demonstration, again making cash more desirable (Dale & Brown, 2007). As a result, actuaries tend to price long-term care insurance policies with cash benefits higher than those with service benefits.

Premium Subsidies for the Low-Income Population and Students

Many government programs provide a subsidy for low-income people. For example, both Medicare and Social Security are financed so that higher-income people pay more than lower-income people; Medicaid does not require low-income people to pay a premium to enroll, and the cost is borne primarily by higher-income people who do not participate in the program. To encourage enrollment in the CLASS program of full-time students and people with incomes below the federal poverty level who work, premiums for these groups were to be only $5 per month, far below the expected premiums for the nonsubsidized population. These premium subsidies, however, were to be financed equally by all other insurance enrollees, not by federal general revenues. As a result, the subsidy for low-income workers and full-time students would have substantially raised premiums for people not in those categories. The SCAN Foundation/Avalere Health premium simulator estimates that premiums for a policy with this type of low-income subsidy would have been about 50% higher than the premiums would have been without a low-income subsidy (SCAN Foundation/Avalere Health, 2010). The prescription drug benefit in the Medicare Catastrophic Coverage Act, which was to be financed entirely by Medicare beneficiaries, encountered the same problem (Oliver, Lee, & Lipton, 2004).

OTHER IMPLEMENTATION ISSUES

Although the CLASS Act will not be implemented as enacted, it raised several implementation issues that must be addressed by any public long-term care insurance program (Nadash, Doty, Mahoney, & Von Schwanenflugel, 2012). These implementation issues include how to pay for administrative costs; what should be the benefit triggers; how eligibility for benefits should be determined; what the link between disability and benefit levels is; if provided, whether there should be restrictions on the use of cash benefits; how to market a voluntary program; and the relationship between public and private long-term care insurance.

Administrative Costs

Financing for CLASS Act benefits was to be entirely from premiums paid by enrollees. No more than 3% of the premiums were to be used to pay for administrative expenses, which is substantially below the 30% to 40% of premiums that is typical for individually purchased private long-term care insurance. Although in line with administrative expenses for Medicare, 3% of premium would have been problematic for a voluntary program, especially during the early years, when marketing the plan to workers and employers would have been critical for its success. However, as noted above, nothing in the statute precludes additional administrative expenses from being funded through government appropriations if Congress and the president agree to do so.

Benefit Thresholds

The ACA specifies that the Secretary of the U.S. Department of Health and Human Services had to set an eligibility standard for the receipt of benefits that included (1) limitation in at least two or three of six activities of daily living (ADLs), (2) requiring substantial supervision to protect an individual from threats to personal safety because of cognitive impairment, or (3) an impairment equivalent to these two disability levels. These standards closely follow those established for tax-qualified private long-term care insurance under the Health Insurance Portability and Accountability Act of 1997 (Cohen, Gordon, & Miller, 2011). The Secretary's choice of eligibility criteria, especially in the choice of the minimum number of ADL limitations, would have involved a trade off between covering more people with long-term care needs but with higher insurance premiums versus covering fewer people but with lower insurance premiums.

If equity is to be maintained, then the eligibility standard across the three criteria needs to identify people with roughly the same level of service need. This may be difficult. For example, using Channeling Demonstration data, Spector and Kemper (1994) found that people with cognitive impairment but no ADL needs used 20% fewer formal and informal care hours than persons with two ADL limitations without cognitive impairment. The challenge is to develop an equitable cutpoint to receive benefits that accounts for interactions between physical and cognitive impairment.

The third eligibility standard, impairment equivalent to the ADL and cognitive impairment standards, is thought by most observers to be designed to include people with intellectual disabilities and some people with severe mental illness who need long-term care services. Although these two populations receive substantial amounts of Medicaid services, these groups rarely are covered by private long-term care insurance policies, and there is little experience with serving this population through an insurance mechanism.

Benefit Eligibility Determination

The legislation requires the establishment of an "eligibility assessment system," which would have determined whether "an individual has a functional limitation, as certified by a licensed health care practitioner" that qualifies for benefits. One possibility is to establish a benefit eligibility determination process that relies heavily on documentation provided by the enrollee's medical provider, an approach similar to cash disability insurance programs such as the Social Security Disability Insurance program. However, functional assessments are rarely included in medical records, and physicians lack expertise in conducting such assessments. Moreover, it seems unlikely that a consistent and uniform approach to assessment would be possible using beneficiary providers, creating horizontal equity issues. In addition, medical providers would have little incentive not to certify individuals as meeting the criteria, potentially increasing the number of people receiving benefits improperly.

An alternative approach would have independent or insurance program staff conduct functional assessments, as is typically done with private long-term care insurance (Gordon, Cohen, & Miller, 2011) and with the Medicaid program when determining the need for long-term care services (Tucker & Kelley, 2011a, 2011b). Japan, Germany, and the Netherlands all depend on these types of independent functional assessments as a way to ensure that only people who meet the eligibility criteria receive benefits (Campbell et al., 2010; Nadash et al., 2012; Wiener, Tilly, & Cuellar, 2003). In implementing a separate assessment service, the CLASS program would have needed to hire or contract with assessors, establish an assessment instrument, develop detailed instructions for conducting the assessment, conduct trainings, and create data reporting and service authorization systems.

Benefit Size, Accountability, and Restrictions on Use

Benefits under the CLASS insurance program were to be cash rather than a specific set of covered services. Receipt of this money would not have affected eligibility for government programs, such as Medicaid and Supplemental Security Income, and would not have been considered income for tax purposes. The benefit was designed primarily to cover home- and community-based services, although it could be used to pay for nursing home or residential care. As such, the benefit was consciously designed to shift the balance of care away from institutional care and toward home- and community-based services.

The cash payment amount, which would have been set by the secretary, initially would have averaged at least $50 per day and would have varied by level of need. Beneficiaries with a higher level of need would have received a higher payment than those with lesser needs. Thus, hypothetically, people with two ADL deficits could have received a benefit of $30 a day, while people with four ADL deficits could have received a benefit of $70 a day, so long as the average of all people receiving payments was $50 a day. Even at higher levels of disability, the payment level was unlikely to be enough to cover the cost of nursing home care. The benefit amount would have increased annually by the Consumer Price Index to cope with inflation over time. Beneficiaries who used their allowance to hire workers would have had to pay Social Security and Medicare taxes as well as federal and state unemployment taxes on their employees' behalf.

Although the average $50-per-day benefit payment level was criticized as inadequate, it was to be paid every day that the individuals qualified for benefits regardless of whether they used services on that day. Many people receiving paid home care do not receive it every day. Moreover, $50 a day

($18,250 a year) is about twice what Medicaid spends per year on participants in home- and community-based services waiver programs for older people and younger persons with physical disabilities (Ng, Harrington, & O'Malley, 2009). In addition, the amount compares favorably to cash home care benefits in several European countries (Nadash et al., 2011).

The legislation specified that the secretary would have to establish between two and six benefit levels but does not mandate a specific number or what the cash benefits would have been for each level. Germany established three basic benefit levels based on disability levels for its public long-term care insurance program, which accounts for hours of care and the frequency of care needed. Although Japan's long-term care insurance program does not provide a cash benefit, it has seven disability levels with a maximum allowable insurance expenditure for individuals at each level (Campbell et al., 2010).

Converting different levels of disability to a cash payment would have required analyses of service use and assumptions about what types of care are needed at each level of disability. Earlier studies of Channeling Demonstration data by Spector and Kemper (1994) found wide variations in service use within the same disability level. Implementation of the CLASS Act might have drawn on the experience of state Medicaid programs, which routinely link levels of need to specific expenditure levels as part of the service planning process.

Despite the legislation's repeated references to a "cash benefit," the statute is ambiguous about whether beneficiaries would have had unlimited freedom regarding how the money could be used. In Germany's long-term care insurance program, the cash benefits can be used for whatever the beneficiary would like. This approach maximizes the ability of individuals to meet their unique long-term care needs and would make the benefit more akin to the Social Security disability benefit, but it also increases the likelihood that the funds will be used for other than long-term care purposes.

In contrast, in England and the Netherlands and in Medicaid participant direction programs in the United States, beneficiaries may use the funds to purchase a very wide range of services and supports, but they must spend the funds on long-term care broadly defined (Nadash et al., 2011; Wiener et al., 2003). Restrictions on what the funds may be used for and the statutory requirement for documentation of expenditures may lessen concerns about improper use of the funds, but such requirements would increase administrative expenses for the program and administrative burdens for beneficiaries unless funds are routinely handled by third-party fiscal agents.

Marketing

Because enrollment in CLASS was to be voluntary, the program would have needed to actively market to potential enrollees, a task that would have been difficult and costly. Moreover, because most government programs are free to users, the federal government does not have extensive experience in marketing programs that require voluntary enrollment and substantial fees, although the Office of Personnel Management does manage the Federal Long-Term Care Insurance Program for federal employees, and the Department of Health and Human Services sponsored the Own Your Future campaign, which sought to encourage people to plan for their own long-term care needs. The campaign included a letter signed by the governor in each participating state, a state-specific planning kit, and a state-funded media campaign (Long Term Care Group, Inc., & LifePlans, Inc., 2006). In addition, the government has experience marketing enlistment in the military, smoking cessation, and AIDS prevention.

Marketing private long-term care insurance has always been difficult because of the incorrect belief that Medicare or standard health insurance covers long-term care, the denial or lack of knowledge about the risk of needing long-term care, and the high cost of policies (LifePlans, Inc., 2007). All of these factors would have applied to potential purchasers of the CLASS insurance product. Moreover, although non-buyers of long-term care insurance typically have a high level of mistrust of private insurers, the public's overall trust in the federal government is also at a low level. In a spring 2011 survey by the Pew Research Center for the People & the Press, 69% of respondents reported that they trust the government only some of the time or never (Pew Research Center for the People & the Press, 2011). Strong supporters of the role of government, perhaps single-payer advocates, might have formed a core group willing to enroll in CLASS.

Another major marketing barrier would have been the affordability of CLASS, which also has been a major obstacle to the purchase of private long-term care insurance (Wiener et al., 1994). In a survey of residents of Hawaii in 2010, 55% of respondents favored the CLASS Act and 20% indicated an interest in enrolling, but only 3% expressed a willingness to pay $80 or more per month for the insurance, much less than most premium estimates (Khatutsky, Wiener, Best, & McMichael, 2011). Thus, although respondents in Hawaii found the concept of a voluntary public long-term care insurance program appealing, they were not willing to spend the money necessary to enroll.

Relationship Between CLASS and Private Long-Term Care Insurance

By expanding the government role, the CLASS Act likely would have supplanted private long-term care insurance to some extent, although it would have increased the overall number of people who would have had long-term care insurance. Despite this direct competition, the CLASS Act deliberately left a substantial role for private long-term care insurance. The CLASS Act was designed to provide only a basic benefit, not comprehensive coverage, for long-term care. In particular, CLASS insurance benefits would not have been enough to pay the costs of nursing home care. As a result, private insurers would have had the option to offer wraparound benefits to the CLASS insurance plan, somewhat analogous to how private insurers provide supplemental coverage for Medicare. Indeed, some CLASS Act advocates argued that by better defining the need for long-term care coverage, the CLASS Act would have increased demand for private long-term care insurance. The insurance industry was skeptical of this argument and never embraced that role.

CONCLUSIONS

Inclusion of the CLASS Act in the final health care reform legislation was a surprise to many long-term care experts and advocates. Widespread consensus exists among both liberals and conservatives on the need to reduce reliance on institutional care and provide more home- and community-based services and to give people with disabilities greater control over their services. However, little consensus exists on long-term care financing reform. States that have been active in delivery system reform have been silent on restructuring financing. Although Hawaii and Washington State debated public long-term care insurance programs over the past decade, neither state enacted a program. At the national level, little discussion of long-term care financing reform has occurred since the failure of the Clinton health care reform proposals in 1994 (Wiener, Estes, Goldenson, & Goldberg, 2001). Indeed, to the extent that there has been any debate at all, it has focused on ways to promote private long-term care insurance.

The CLASS Act legislation did not address the long-term care needs of the population currently retired or those unable to work. Over the long run, however, the CLASS Act had as its goal to shift the financing system from one based primarily on Medicaid to one based on insurance principles where risks are spread broadly among the insured. Because initial enrollment was to be limited to people in the workforce, this transformation would have been a slow process at best. Even for workers in their 50s, it would have been another 25 or 30 years or more before many would start using long-term care.

With the decision not to implement CLASS as written, what now for the program and for long-term care financing? As of this writing in December 2011, opponents of health care reform and of the idea of a public long-term care insurance program are pushing for repeal of the legislation, while CLASS Act supporters and advocates of an increased role for public programs are proposing modifications to CLASS that would address the structural problems of the program.

The goals of modifications to CLASS would be to reduce the risk of adverse selection and to drastically lower the premium. Within the framework of a voluntary public insurance program self-financed by participants, changes could include tightening the work requirement, reducing the benefit from lifetime to some shorter period of time, limiting use of the cash benefit to long-term care services and supports, and eliminating the low-income and student subsidy. Although these changes would undoubtedly reduce the premiums, they would also make the program look a lot more like private insurance. With these modifications, there would be no element of making the program more affordable to low-income people, and all but a few younger adults with disabilities would be prevented from participating. Younger adults with disabilities would also lose out with a shorter benefit period and a more restrictive cash benefit. Although not its intention, "fixing" CLASS would likely mean making it into a program that works best for older people with relatively short periods of need. The revised program would offer little for younger adults with disabilities. The addition of general tax revenues could also alleviate many of these problems but would be extremely difficult to obtain in the current political environment. Indeed, even legislative passage of modifications of CLASS is difficult to imagine in the current political environment.

Even with these changes, the question remains whether adverse selection would be adequately addressed and the premiums made low enough to be affordable to large numbers of people. Mandatory enrollment and progressive tax financing would solve those problems and allow the program to meet the social policy goals of providing coverage for younger adults with disabilities and subsidies for low-income people, but these solutions face very large political and fiscal barriers that make their enactment unlikely.

Although CLASS held out the promise of a different long-term care financing system, the United States is back to where it has been over the last 45 years: a financing system dominated by Medicaid and catastrophic out-of-pocket costs with little hope for a robust private long-term care insurance market. Although long-term care is not to blame, Medicaid is under intense financial pressure at the state and federal levels and there is great resistance to higher spending.

With the aging of the population, the number of people needing long-term care is sure to increase dramatically, and with it the need for additional long-term care services and expenditures. The number of older people with disabilities is projected to double between 2000 and 2030 (Johnson, Toohey, & Wiener, 2007). Even under the current system, public expenditures for long-term care as a percentage of the gross domestic product are projected to double or triple by 2050 (Martins, de la Maisonneuve, & Bjørnerud, 2006). One thing is certain. There is no way to finance services for twice as many people for the same percentage of the economy as we have now. Somehow the United States needs to find a way to bring additional financing into the long-term care system. The unpalatable alternative is to reduce the already inadequate quantity and quality of services for people with disabilities of all ages.

REFERENCES

American Academy of Actuaries. (2009). *Re: Actuarial issues and policy implications of a federal long-term care insurance program.* Washington, DC: Author. Retrieved from http://www.actuary.org/pdf/health/class_july09.pdf

American Association for Long-Term Care Insurance. (2010). *The 2010 sourcebook for long-term care insurance information.* Westlake Village, CA: Author.

Campbell, J. C., Ikegami, N., & Gibson, M. J. (2010). Lessons from public long-term care insurance in Germany and Japan. *Health Affairs, 29*(1), 87–95. Retrieved from http://content.healthaffairs.org/cgi/reprint/29/1/87

Cohen, M. A., Gordon, J., & Miller, J. (2011). *The historical development of benefit eligibility triggers underlying the CLASS plan.* Long Beach, CA: The SCAN Foundation. Retrieved from http://www.thescanfoundation.org/sites/default/files/TSF_CLASS_TA_No2_History_Benefit_Eligibility_FINAL.pdf

Dale, S. B., & Brown, R. S. (2007). How does cash and counseling affect costs? *Health Services Research, 42*(1, Part II), 488–509.

Eiken, S., Kate, K., Burwell, B., & Gold, L. (2010). *Medicaid long-term care expenditures, FY 2009.* Cambridge, MA: Thomson Reuters.

Feder, J., Komisar, H., & Friedland, R. (2007). *Long-term care financing: Policy options for the future.* Washington, DC: Georgetown University. Retrieved from http://ltc.georgetown.edu/forum/ltcfinalpaper061107.pdf

Foster, R. (2010). *Estimated financial effects of the Patient Protection and Affordable Care Act, as amended.* Baltimore, MD: Centers for Medicare & Medicaid Services.

Genworth Financial. (2010). *Genworth 2010 cost of care survey.* Richmond, VA: Author. Retrieved from http://www.genworth.com/content/etc/medialib/genworth_v2/pdf/ltc_cost_of_care.Par.14625.File.dat/2010_Cost_of_Care_Survey_Full_Report.pdf

Gibson, M. J., & Redfoot, D. L. (2007). *Comparing long-term care in Germany and the United States: What can we learn from each other?* Washington, DC: AARP. Retrieved from http://assets.aarp.org/rgcenter/il/2007_19_usgerman_ltc.pdf

Gordon, J., Cohen, M. A., & Miller, J. (2011). *The independent in-person assessment process.* Long Beach, CA: The SCAN Foundation. Retrieved from http://www.thescanfoundation.org/sites/default/files/TSF_CLASS_TA_No_4_LTCI_Assessment_FINAL_0.pdf

Greenlee, K. (2011). *Memorandum on the CLASS program to Secretary Sebelius.* Washington, DC: U.S. Department of Health and Human Services. Retrieved from http://aspe.hhs.gov/daltcp/reports/2011/class/CLASSmemo.pdf

Johnson, R. W., & Park, J. S. (2011). *Who purchases long-term care insurance?* Washington, DC: The Urban Institute. Retrieved from http://www.urban.org/uploadedpdf/412324-Long-Term-Care-Insurance.pdf

Johnson, R. W., Toohey, D., & Wiener, J. M. (2007). *Meeting the long-term care needs of the baby boomers: How changing families will affect paid helpers and institutions.* Washington, DC: The Urban Institute. Retrieved from http://www.urban.org/publications/311451.html

Kaye, H. S. (2010). The impact of the 2007–2009 recession on workers with disabilities. *Monthly Labor Review, 133*(10), 19–30.

Khatutsky, G., Wiener, J. M., Best, H., & McMichael, J. (2011). *Assessing long-term care policy options in Hawaii: Results from the Hawaii long-term care survey.* Honolulu, HI: The Hawaii Long-Term Care Commission. Retrieved from http://www.publicpolicycenter.hawaii.edu/documents/RTI-Survey_Results_Report-FINAL.pdf

LifePlans, Inc. (2007). *Who buys long-term care insurance? A 15-year study of buyers and non-buyers, 1990–2005.* Washington, DC: America's Health Insurance Plans. Retrieved from http://www.ahip.org/content/default.aspx?bc=39|341|328|21022

Long Term Care Group, Inc., & LifePlans, Inc. (2006). *Final report on the "Own Your Future" consumer survey.* Washington, DC: Office of the Assistant Secretary for Policy and Evaluation, U.S. Department of Health and Human Services.

Madrian, B. C., & Shea, D. F. (2000). The power of suggestion: Inertia in 401(k) participation and savings behavior. *Quarterly Journal of Economics, 116*(4), 1149–1187.

Martins, J. O., de la Maisonneuve, C., & Bjørnerud, S. (2006). *Projecting OECD health and long-term care expenditures: What are the main drivers?* Paris: Organization for Economic Co-Operation and Development.

Merlis, M. (2003). *Private long-term care insurance: Who should buy it and what should they buy?* Washington, DC: Kaiser Family Foundation.

Miller, E. A. (2011). Flying beneath the radar of health reform: The Community Living Assistance Services and Supports (CLASS) Act. *Gerontologist, 51*(2), 145–155.

Munnell, A. H., & Hurwitz, J. (2011). *What is "CLASS" and will it work?* Boston, MA: Center for Retirement Research at Boston College. Retrieved from http://crr.bc.edu/images/stories/Briefs/IB_11-3.pdf

Nadash, P., Doty, P., Mahoney, K. J., & Von Schwanenflugel, M. (2012). European long-term care programs: Lessons for community living assistance services and supports? *Health Services Research, 47*(1), 309–328.

Ng, T., Harrington, C., & O'Malley, M. (2009). *Medicaid home and community-based service programs: Data update.* Washington, DC: Kaiser Family Foundation. Retrieved from http://www.kff.org/medicaid/upload/7720-03.pdf

Oliver, T. R., Lee, P. R., & Lipton, H. L. (2004). A political history of Medicare and prescription drug coverage. *The Milbank Quarterly, 82*(2), 283–354.

Pew Research Center for the People & the Press. (2011). *Fewer are angry at government, but discontent remains high.* Washington, DC: Author. Retrieved from http://people-press.org/2011/03/03/fewer-are-angry-at-government-but-discontent-remains-high/

Sebelius, K. (2011). *Letter to Congress about CLASS.* Washington, DC: U.S. Department of Health and Human Services. Retrieved from http://www.hhs.gov/secretary/letter10142011.html

SCAN Foundation/Avalere Health. (2010). *Long-term care policy simulato.* Los Angeles, CA: Author. Retrieved from http://www.ltcpolicysimulator.org/

Spector, W. D., & Kemper, P. (1994). Disability and cognitive impairment criteria: Targeting those who need the most home care. *Gerontologist*, *34*(5), 640–651.

Tucker, S. M., & Kelley, M. E. (2011a). *Elements of a functional assessment for Medicaid personal care services*. Long Beach, CA: The SCAN Foundation. Retrieved from http://www.thescanfoundation.org/sites/default/files/TSF_CLASS_TA_No_5_Medicaid_Assessment_FINAL.pdf

Tucker, S. M., & Kelley, M. E. (2011b). *Functional assessment processes for Medicaid personal care services*. Long Beach, CA: The SCAN Foundation. Retrieved from http://www.thescanfoundation.org/sites/default/files/TSF_CLASS_TA_No_7_Medicaid_Assessment_Process_FINAL.pdf

Tumlinson, A., Aguiar, C., & Watts, M. O. (2009). *Closing the long-term care funding gap: The challenge of private long-term care insurance*. Washington, DC: Kaiser Family Foundation. Retrieved from http://www.kff.org/insurance/upload/Closing-the-Long-Term-Care-Funding-Gap-The-Challenge-of-Private-Long-Term-Care-Insurance-Report.pdf

U.S. Census Bureau. (2010). *Median earnings in the last 12 months (in 2009 inflation adjusted dollars) by disability status by sex for the civilian non-institutionalized population age 16 years and over with earnings*. Hyattsville, MD: Author. Retrieved from http://factfinder.census.gov/servlet/DTTable?_bm=y&-geo_id=01000US&-ds_name=ACS_2009_1YR_G00_&-SubjectID=18599106&-_lang=en&-mt_name=ACS_2009_1YR_G2000_B18140&-format=&-CONTEXT=dt

U.S. Congressional Budget Office. (2010, March 20). *Letter from Douglas Elmendorf, Director of the Congressional Budget Office, to Speaker Nancy Pelosi, House of Representatives*. Washington, DC: Author. Retrieved from http://www.cbo.gov/ftpdocs/113xx/doc11355/hr4872.pdf

U.S. Department of Health and Human Services. (2011). *A report on the actuarial, marketing and legal analyses of the CLASS program*. Washington, DC: Author. Retrieved from http://aspe.hhs.gov/daltcp/reports/2011/class/index.pdf

U.S. Office of Personnel Management. (2011). *FLTCIP premiums calculator*. Washington, DC: Author. Retrieved from https://www.ltcfeds.com/ltcWeb/do/assessing_your_needs/ratecalcOut

Walker, L., & Accius, J. (2010). *Access to long-term services and supports: A 50-state survey of Medicaid financial eligibility standards*. Washington, DC: AARP.

Wiener, J. M., Estes, C. L., Goldenson, S. M., & Goldberg, S. C. (2001). What happened to long-term care in the health reform debate of 1993–1994? Lessons for the future. *The Milbank Quarterly*, *79*(2), 207–252.

Wiener, J. M., Illston, L. H., & Hanley, R. J. (1994). *Sharing the burden: Strategies for public and private long-term care insurance*. Washington, DC: The Brookings Institution.

Wiener, J. M., & Sullivan, C. M. (1995). Long-term care for the younger population: A policy synthesis. In J. M. Wiener, S. B. Clauser, & D. L. Kennell (Eds.), *Persons with disabilities: Issues in health financing and service delivery* (pp. 291–324). Washington, DC: The Brookings Institution.

Wiener, J. M., Tilly, J., & Cuellar, A. E. (2003). *Consumer-directed home care in the Netherlands, Germany and England*. Washington, DC: AARP. Retrieved from http://assets.aarp.org/rgcenter/health/2003_12_eu_cd.pdf

A 10-Foot Rope for a 50-Yard Drop: The CLASS Act in the Patient Protection and Affordable Care Act

WILLIAM G. WEISSERT, PhD

Professor, Florida State University, and Director, Masters of Public Health;
Faculty Associate, Pepper Institute on Aging & Public Policy,
Florida State University, Tallahassee, Florida, USA, and
Professor Emeritus, University of Michigan, Ann Arbor, Michigan, USA

The Community Living Assistance Services and Supports (CLASS) Act, part of the 2010 health care reform, would have paid a daily cash payment toward the costs of long-term care. This article points out that although the CLASS Act may have been sufficient to cover the costs of most home- and community-based services, it was an inadequate response to the most pressing long-term care financing problem facing baby boomers: nursing home care costs. The risk of needing a nursing home is higher than other catastrophic risks. Boomers lack savings to pay those costs. CLASS aimed to encourage people to use home- and community-based services to substitute for nursing home care, but research spanning decades shows there is little substitution effect.

INTRODUCTION

Picture this: Your house has burned down, you still owe the mortgage, and the finance company wants its monthly payment; your car was in the garage so it burned too as did all your clothes and belongings; your health insurance premiums and co-payments are both going up; and by the way, you were already unemployed. Your insurance company offers you $50 a day. Are you happy?

Of course you're not. Likewise, an 80-year-old widow who needs a nursing home costing $6,000 to $7,000 a month who's offered $1,500 a month to pay for it is not going to get into a quality home; not going to avoid making herself destitute to go on Medicaid; not going to be in a position to do much about the inadequate staffing, uneven facility quality, weak regulatory enforcement, and lack of competition in the nursing home market for Medicaid patients; and not going to be able to do much about the lack of choices she'll face in that market. The nursing home industry has long been burdened by a bad reputation (Kaiser Family Foundation, 2007; Miller, Mor, & Clark, 2010), much of it earned with deficiencies, patient safety violations, and insufficient government oversight (Castle, Wagner, Ferguson, & Handler, 2011; Harrington, 2002). Homes that serve primarily Medicaid patients are of particular concern, as Mor et al. and others have shown (Mor, Zinn, Angelelli, Teno, & Miller, 2004; Castle & Ferguson, 2011). Homes that serve the poor tend to be non–hospital-affiliated, understaffed, resource-constrained by low occupancy and low payment rates, and located in poor counties where African Americans are disproportionately represented. Forgive our widow if she is a bit confused by how the Community Living Assistance Services and Supports (CLASS) Act was going to fix these nursing home quality and financing problems for her.

THE CLASS ACT, FEATURES, AND FLAWS

No, the CLASS Act was not going to help her. Nor was it intended to. The CLASS Act that passed as part of the Patient Protection and Affordable Cost Act (PPACA; Section 8002 of PPACA, amending the Public Health Service Act by adding Title XXXIII) was in no significant way the answer to one of the nation's most vexing problems: how to finance long-term care, and with that financing, how to bring "class" to a system long known for its varying standards of care. CLASS was instead a specialized disability payment—replete with substantial potential for adverse selection and moral hazard—intended to expand use of home- and community-based care, not nursing home care (Miller, 2011; Meiners, 2011).

CLASS, had the Obama administration not stopped implementation due to its fatal design flaws, would have provided a modest daily benefit to disabled individuals who had bought into the voluntary long-term care insurance program. It would have paid a minimum average cash benefit of $50 per day, scaled to level of functional dependence. Buyers were required to work at minimal levels for 3 years (earning $1,120 in 2011) to qualify for benefits. Premiums were to vary only by age; no underwriting based on current or future projected disability was to take place, although full-time working students aged 18 to 22 years and those with incomes below the poverty level would have paid nominal premiums only (~$5 per month). Benefits could not start until 5 years after initial purchase. But once benefits began, they could have lasted the rest of one's life. With little to discourage the already disabled from purchasing the insurance, it would have become an unattractive option for people who want insurance against future risk but are at present disability-free. They could do better in a private market comprising mostly low-risk people because private vendors screen for preexisting conditions to keep costs down.

The legislation, thanks to a Republican-sponsored amendment, precluded the CLASS program from drawing revenue from the general federal treasury; instead, it was to be financed entirely by member premiums. Initial premiums were to be set to ensure 75 years of program solvency; subsequently, premiums could be adjusted if the program's fiscal situation had changed over a 20-year time horizon. Administrative costs were capped at 3% of premiums paid. As such, unless Congress allocated additional appropriations there would have been few resources with which to market the program to attract better-off risks or to institute mechanisms to prevent fraud and abuse, a legitimate concern in consumer-directed cash programs (Miller, 2011). Criticisms of the act focused heavily on the potential for adverse selection, both conceptually before it passed (American Academy of Actuaries, 2009) and again after it became law (Miller, 2011; Shesgreen, 2011; Wiener, 2010). Even Secretary Sebelius called the CLASS Act unsustainable (Pear, 2011).

FOCUS OF THIS ARTICLE

Here we focus on what may be this legislation's most important shortcoming: failure to acknowledge the costs of nursing home care, clearly the most important risk for seniors as they age. This risk was not well addressed by the modest cash benefit of the CLASS Act. The article also reprises the many research findings showing that expansion of home care services would not obviate the need for nursing home care, strongly suggesting that a long-term care insurance program that neglects the risk for nursing home placement is necessarily incomplete. CLASS may have encouraged disability claims through the provision of a cash payment to relatives and friends to perform caregiving as authorized under the Act. And it might have discouraged Congress from further addressing the unmet need of nursing home financing under the mistaken belief that it had done so already.

NOT SOLD AS NURSING HOME INSURANCE,
BUT POSSIBLE CONFUSION

"Long-term care" is a confusing term to many people. A MetLife survey in 2009 found that nearly one-third of respondents thought it was anything from hospital care to chemotherapy (Moeller, 2009). Furthermore, most of those responding equated long-term care with nursing homes rather than home- and community-based services. Given that a large proportion of commentators, blogs, news reports, and other sources referred to the CLASS Act as "long-term care insurance," both when it was being considered as part of health reform and after its passage, many people may have believed that the reform bill covered the full cost of nursing home services (Pickert, 2009; Elder Guru, n.d.; Koff, 2010). It would not have paid enough to accomplish that goal, however. It primarily covered services delivered at home or in the community, including, potentially, a significant portion of the cost of assisted living.

COVERS HOME CARE, RELIEVES CAREGIVERS, BUT LITTLE
FOR NURSING HOME COSTS

There is much to recommend a program that pays for home- and community-based services to non-aged adults with disabilities and frail and disabled elders. Formal services can provide relief to overburdened daughters and daughters-in-law, the primary providers of unpaid, informal care for this ballooning population of needy Americans (National Alliance for Caregiving, 2009). Home care has been shown to improve the life satisfaction of caregivers in particular and to a lesser, and sometimes more fleeting, degree, the life satisfaction of some patients (Doty, 2010; Grabowski, 2006; Weissert & Hedrick, 1994; Weissert, Cready, & Pawelak, 1988). Caregivers of adults—the sizeable army of at least 13 million people quietly providing free care day and night—are themselves known to suffer a burden: stress, loss of sleep and income, pension losses, job difficulties, and self-doubt about their ability to do caregiving—especially therapies—properly (MetLife Mature Market Institute, 1999, 2011). Business losses are substantial due to distracted workers and the need to replace those who give up their jobs to become full-time caregivers (Genworth Life Insurance Company, 2010).

But those who can use home- and community-based care tend not to be nursing home candidates or patients, even without home care. Their disabilities are not typical of nursing home residents. Although there may be some degree of overlap, the two services appeal primarily to different populations. This conclusion is reflected in the many studies examining expansion of home care benefits (Weissert & Hedrick, 1994; Weissert et al., 1988). Control groups in those studies were similar in characteristics to the experimental groups but received no expanded home care benefits. Even though the vast majority could have qualified for nursing home admission, most did not enter nursing homes. They stayed out regardless of whether they received home care because care and cost demands, even in the absence of additional home care services, did not necessitate placement.

This finding is important because it points to a policy choice underlying the CLASS Act. The needs of the caregiving population and the lesser-impaired dependent population were dealt with by this program before anyone addressed the crushing needs of the millions of Americans who will face nursing home admission in an overburdened, underfunded, and expensive system of uneven quality. The nursing home care system is bankrupting states as they struggle to pay their long-term care costs. States would have gotten little relief from the CLASS Act.

The CLASS Act entitled the recipients to a cash payment for each day they qualified as disabled. By the terms of the act, a person would have had to have been brought into the program before retirement, hold it for 5 years (working very minimally for at least 3 of those), and meet standards not yet set by the Secretary of the U.S. Department of Health and Human Services for qualifying for benefits based on physical limitations, mental impairment, or some combination equivalent to limitations in two, perhaps three, activities of daily living (ADLs).

Contrast this relatively low level of impairment with the 74% of nursing home patients who experience limitations in three or more of the traditional five ADLs: bathing, dressing, toileting, eating, and transferring, either from bed to chair or chair to bed (National Center for Health Statistics, 2002). The ADL scale is progressive: Those who need help with bathing and dressing are still pretty much self-reliant and mobile. Those who need help eating are typically able to perform few or none of the other functions in the scale, and they are almost certainly immobilized and heavily dependent on human help (Katz, 1972). Thus, not only are nursing home residents characterized by limitations in more ADLs but they have losses in more advanced ADLs, indicating greater frailty and disability.

Moreover, many nursing home patients experience some sort of mental illness, dementia, disorientation, or behavior problem and are likely to be close to 80 years old at admission, with barely one in five having a living spouse (National Center for Health Statistics, 2002). In contrast, more than three-fourths of community-dwelling elders are married to a living spouse, and greater than 70% of younger disabled people are likely to be married.

So people who would have qualified for care under the CLASS Act would not usually have been people at high risk for nursing home placement. We know from studies of home care that despite screening to limit enrollment of people who would have nominally qualified for nursing home care in many states, most of those who enrolled would never have actually entered nursing homes, regardless of whether they received home care

(Doty, 2010; Grabowski, 2006; Weissert & Hedrick, 1994; Weissert et al., 1988). Their personal, physical, mental, and social resources would have kept them out. And if they did receive home care, it would have had very little effect on most people's need for eventual nursing home placement (Miller & Weissert, 2000).

In other words, home care has yet to be proven a significant factor in keeping people at home despite a plethora of studies seeking to show that effect. It simply is not very effective both because most of those who use home care are not at high risk for going to nursing homes and because home care has limited ability to mitigate the factors that place people in nursing homes: age, functional dependence, bowel incontinence, cognitive impairment, combinations of mental and physical impairment, and most of all, prior nursing home use (Friedman, Steinwachs, Rathouz, Burton, & Mukamel, 2005; Gaugler, Duval, Anderson, & Kane, 2007; Liu, Coughlin, & McBride, 1991). Loneliness, or at least extreme loneliness, has sometimes been suggested as a contributing factor to nursing home admission, although much less often than the factors listed above. Perhaps this is one factor that home care does help mitigate and may explain how home care does have small effects on nursing home use (Russell, Curtona, de la Mora, & Wallace, 1997; Coughlin, Timothy, McBride, & Liu, 1990), although rarely enough to produce net financial savings (Doty, 2010; Grabowski, 2006; Weissert & Hedrick, 1994; Weissert et al., 1988). Kemper, Applebaum, and Harrigan (1987) summed up the problem this way: "Small reductions in nursing home costs for some [clients] are more than offset by the increased costs of providing expanded community services to others who, even without expanded services, would not enter nursing homes." For most users of home care, the service will be a complement to nursing home use, not a substitute.

INABILITY TO PAY FOR NURSING HOME CARE

Americans are most worried about their ability to pay for their retirement (Mendes, 2010), and they should be. They are in very poor shape when it comes to retirement finances. The Employee Benefits Research Institute (EBRI; 2010) estimates that the average retiree has little savings to pay for retirement, and none to pay for nursing home care. EBRI's survey of workers showed that 27% have saved less than $1,000 and 54% had saved less than $25,000 (Helman, Copeland, & VanDerhei, 2010). That is just over half of one year's income ($47,400 in 2010) for the average American wage earner (United States Central Intelligence Agency, 2010) and barely a third of the cost of a year in a nursing home (Genworth Life Insurance Company, 2011). But EBRI also estimates that Medicare co-payments are due to rise significantly, leaving baby boomers very short of funds to cover other health care expenditures (EBRI, 2010). Since only about 10% of people older than

65 buy long-term care insurance (Weiner, 2010) and since the values of their homes—where most baby boomers have traditionally stored much of their net worth—have fallen to the point that 15 million homeowners owe larger mortgages than their homes are worth and another 5 million have been lost to foreclosure since 2006 (Elphinstone, 2010), there is very little prospect that baby boomers will be able to pay for nursing home care when the time comes.

The Congressional Budget Office estimated that participating in the CLASS Act would have cost enrollees as much as $123 a month for the rest of their lives (Elmendorf, 2009) and probably considerably more if adverse selection occurred and a disproportionate number of high-risk individuals chose to enroll (American Academy of Actuaries, 2009). And if the CLASS Act payment did not cover all the costs of home care, additional patient or family funds would have been needed. What would this mean for a patient's ability to pay for nursing home care when the need arose some 5 or more years after home care started? It would have likely entailed a participant having even fewer resources available to pay privately for nursing home care. The result would have been "spending down" to Medicaid earlier and more public spending.

LONG-TERM CARE INSURANCE RISK, TAKE-UP, AND COSTS

Economists lament the peculiar inability of consumers to discern the difference in the kinds of risks they face between low-cost, high-likelihood risks and high-cost, low-likelihood risks (Pauly, 1990). People tend to want insurance for the things that are very likely to occur but would be affordable out of normal household budgets, but they do not buy insurance for the events that are less likely to occur but catastrophic when they happen. Ironically, with the CLASS Act, the government promoted consumer engagement in just this kind of perverse risk-mitigation behavior. Through automatic workplace enrollment, consumers of all ages would have been encouraged to buy CLASS Act insurance to cover an event that is likely to occur—a modest level of dependency in old age—and for which costs in the way of some home- and community-based care may well be manageable. Moreover, by paying the benefit in cash, the probability of making a claim would likely have been greatly increased because people are more inclined to accept a cash benefit than claim a service-denominated benefit that involves higher personal transactions costs (Spillman, Murtaugh, & Warshawsky, 2003). Yet the same consumer is left virtually naked in the face of the perhaps less likely but financially more devastating need for nursing home care.

In fact, nursing home admission may be a more common occurrence than suggested by calling it "low." Researchers, using a variety of databases and methods across several studies, have estimated the lifetime risk after age 65 of spending time in a nursing home at about 40%, with an expected stay of about 1 year; 20% may stay 5 years or longer; and 2% may stay a decade or more (Murtaugh, Kemper, Spillman, & Carlson, 1997). For many others, the stay will be short, only just preceding death or discharge back to the community. But use is highly skewed when examining length of stay distributions; a very large portion of nursing home use is concentrated in people with long stays. Thus, although 20% of 65-year-olds will spend more than 1 year in a nursing home, 75% of their lifetime use will occur during a stay of longer than 1 year. This suggests an important policy imperative: find a way to lessen the unequal financial burden falling on these long stayers, both on their families and on the state Medicaid programs that pay for them.

Typically, when risk is so catastrophic and so skewed, we look to risk pooling to share the burden. Indeed most people purchase insurance for such catastrophic losses as major car accidents and home fires. Yet risks of those devastating events are estimated to be less than 10% of the risk of needing a nursing home (Long-term Care Insurance Tree, n.d.). Thus, a well-reasoned insurance analysis might suggest that the nation would be well served if we all purchased long-term care insurance to pool our resources against this catastrophic risk. If all 65-year-olds bought into a long-term care insurance pool, average cost would be low given that most would make minimal use due to non-entry or short stays. A 65-year-old buying coverage that pays for a 2-year stay costing about $150 per day with modest inflation protection may pay a premium of $160 per month (The Federal Long-Term Care Insurance Program, n.d.). The premium for a 5-year nursing home stay would be about $250 a month for the average elder buyer. Moreover, most current policies allow trade off of home care days for a fraction of a nursing home day, and the policies pay their own premiums once the patient enters a nursing facility. The CLASS Act failed to include this feature.

Work by Doty, Cohen, Miller, and Shi (2010) showed that 74% of 10 insurance companies' policy holders sampled in their study had filed claims for home care, assisted living, or nursing home residency. Of these, 96% had their claims paid, and the majority were satisfied with their care providers. This suggests that widespread suspicion of long-term care insurance companies and their policies does not appear justified and that generally they seem to render value for money.

If broadly purchased, long-term care insurance would bring in billions of dollars to finance the long-term care used by those who need it. More money could spur higher quality standards due to more competition because insured applicants would be in the market as private-pay patients, and fewer facilities would rely heavily or solely on Medicaid for payment. If instead of the CLASS Act, Congress had mandated automatic enrollment in true long-term care insurance, which, according to the study by Doty et al., would need to cover home care and assisted living along with nursing facility care, the long-term care financing problem might be solved.

Unfortunately, few people realize that they face such high risk of terrible financial loss, and fewer still understand that they are not protected. Surveys show that many people think that their employer's health insurance, Medicare, or Medicaid will kick in to pay their nursing home bills as soon as they need care (e.g., AARP, 2006). They do not understand that neither Medicare nor private health insurance cover much long-term custodial care. Additionally, people do not understand that Medicaid typically does not cover less intensive residential care settings such as assisted living. Furthermore, to receive Medicaid coverage, prospective applicants must spend down almost all of their income and assets. Medicaid kicks in only *after* financial ruin. Taken together, this lack of understanding of the limitations of nursing home coverage provided by private and public health insurance suggests that a systematic, comprehensive education campaign is needed to alert people to these problems. People must realize that while they have insured their homes against loss, they have failed to insure against a much, much greater likelihood of nearly as large a loss due to aging, genetic, and environmental factors. If such a campaign were mounted, people might then seek out long-term care insurance.

On the one hand, many more could afford to purchase long-term care insurance than already do: A tax deduction is available from the federal government as well as some states. On federal tax returns, premium costs can be counted as medical expenses and deducted up to an annual age-adjusted maximum as medical expenses, provided total medical expenses exceed 7.5% of income. On the other hand, this process may be too complicated and restrictive to attract much interest. And there are also those too poor to itemize their deductions or to afford the price of long-term care insurance. For example, in 2006, the average cost at purchase to buyers aged 50 or 70 years was $2,477 and $6,178 per year, respectively (U.S. Government Accountability Office, 2006). Programs to subsidize insurance premiums, perhaps with income adjustments, might prove to be an appropriate and cost-effective approach to addressing the long-term care financing conundrum. Although the Long-Term Care Partnership program was established to boost take-up in the private long-term care insurance market, they exist in only a handful of states and are not widely subscribed (America's Health Insurance Plans, 2007). Moreover, they do not truly subsidize premiums as much as protect assets from the spend-down requirements of Medicaid. A determined program to turn the baby boomers into long-term care insurance buyers is still badly needed.

Unfortunately, instead of expanding access to higher-quality long-term care insurance, baby boomers were given the CLASS Act, a program designed to induce moral hazard in a population that could well have used home care for many years at substantial expense to the risk pool while doing very little to share the burden of the catastrophic risk of nursing home cost that we all face.

THE CLASS ACT AS DISABILITY POLICY

Twenty-five percent of elder Americans are living in the community with one or more limitations in ADLs (Administration on Aging, 2010). We know from studies of disability insurance and Social Security Disability Insurance payment policy that relaxed eligibility for disability payments increases the number of people who report themselves as disabled and increases the number of claimants (Autor & Duggan, 2003). Between 1984 and 2001, there was a 60% increase in disability rolls to 5.3 million Americans despite a general increase in population health. Researchers attribute the increase and an accompanying decline in workforce participation by low-wage workers to less stringent disability screening, lower demand for unskilled workers, and an increase in the payoff for those who make it onto the disability rolls (Autor & Duggan, 2003). The rise in successful claims began its increase with liberalization of Social Security Disability Insurance screening criteria in 1984 and again following passage of the Americans with Disabilities Act in 1990, which resulted in even more liberalized standards for disability claims (Burkhauser & Daly, 2002). It is also speculated that the increasing age at qualification for Social Security retirement benefits will increase the rate of disability claims as well (Burkhauser, Houtenville, & Wittenburg, 2001).

These findings suggest that at least some level of moral hazard would have ensued as disabled people currently coping without assistance came to view themselves as sufficiently in need of assistance to join the CLASS program and make a claim. Assuredly, the 5-year waiting period before an enrollee could start getting paid would have discouraged overuse and, potentially, outright fraud, at least during the program's early years. But it does seem reasonable to ask whether, over time, needy patients in the community would have been encouraged by various vendors, relatives, or others to enroll in the CLASS Act, perhaps have their premiums subsidized by those encouraging enrollment, and then be obligated to turn some or all of their cash benefit over to their premium benefactors for services real or imagined? Estimates suggest that as much as 10% of Medicare and Medicaid program funds may be fraudulently collected, representing an abuse of the system, or are simply waste (Foster, 2009). And these are *vendor* payment programs designed to avoid the problem of paying cash to sick and disabled people. How much of a problem fraud, abuse, and waste would have been if the CLASS Act had been implemented is unknown. But the possibility cannot be dismissed, particularly since the statute limits administrative expenses to no more than 3% of program premiums. Few resources would have been available to program administrators to combat it.

THE CLASS ACT AND NURSING HOME QUALITY

The CLASS Act would not have done much for the myriad of problems faced by those most in need of long-term care: nursing home residents. Low Medicaid payments make it difficult for facilities to provide a high-quality building, retain trained staff, offer amenities, or try to improve patients' quality of life. Competition plays little or no role in the Medicaid market. Patients who can pay privately or are on Medicare are sought after by nursing homes, which improve their facilities and services to attract them. But patients entering on Medicaid or likely to spend down to Medicaid eligibility soon are not attractive to nursing homes, who accept them only to fill beds not filled by private patients. As facilities deteriorate in quality, they make the trade off between the cost of improving their offerings to attract private patients or accepting the lower-paying Medicaid patients who are in no position to demand quality.

In the absence of competition, Medicaid patients must rely on the federal survey and certification process administered by the states to assure that they receive the minimum acceptable level of care. But facilities are rarely denied actual Medicaid certification. Resources for survey and certification are inadequate in most states, and lack of available alternative placements makes it difficult to deny new admissions to facilities found to be in non-compliance (Castle et al., 2011; Harrington, 2002). Rather, facilities found to be providing inadequate care are given opportunities to fix the problems, providing them with limited incentives to avoid the problems in the first place or to let them reoccur after they have been rectified. *Consumer Reports* indicates that facilities on the "bad care" end of its yearly quality list tended to stay there on a recurring or even continuous basis year after year (*Consumer Reports,* 2006). One state's survey and certification director told *Consumer Reports* that addressing problems was sometimes set aside as a priority by nursing facility operators in favor of returning a profit to investors.

The CLASS Act did nothing to fix quality problems in nursing homes, although other provisions of the larger health reform act of which CLASS is but one section call for some improvements in this area. These include greater transparency about ownership, staffing, and expenditures and improvement to the Nursing Home Compare website, which makes quality data public to enhance facility comparisons (Kaiser Family Foundation, n.d.). Unfortunately, comparison sites work only if the consumer has choices. For Medicaid patients, choices are few to none. Typically, they go to the facilities that agree to take them.

CONGRESS AND THE CLASS ACT

In spite of all these limitations, the impact of CLASS on Congress may be the most troublesome consequence of its passage. Congressional agenda scholars know that Congress tends to be loath to take up again an agenda item it feels was completed in a recent Congress (Kingdon, 1995). It is often 10 to 30 years before Congress comes back to a problem considered "solved." The congressional GOP had already put repeal of the CLASS Act on its short priority list for section-by-section repeal of the 2010 health care reform if the party's effort to overturn the entire law fails to bear fruit.

Meanwhile, if reform drags on for a decade or more, the baby boomers will have retired, and in about 2025 and the years following, many of them will begin to need nursing home care. At that point, few will have the resources required to pay for it. Medicaid will most likely be there, groaning under the strain to be certain. Many may wish they had made other plans.

CONCLUSIONS

The CLASS Act was not really addressing long-term care insurance, although it was often referred to as such. It was really a new disability payment program for people who could not typically qualify for existing disability programs. The nominal purpose of the Act was to expand financing for home- and community-based care, an already expanding option under state Medicaid programs despite its limited effectiveness in keeping people out of nursing homes. Because the Act called for cash payments, with few restrictions on how the money could be spent and with strong limits on how much the federal government could spend in administering the program, it may be reasonable to speculate that many of the dollars paid would have simply gone to household expenses, payments to relatives, or whatever else the recipient or her or his guardian decided to spend the money on. Premiums seemed likely to result in a drain on patients' financial resources, thereby increasing the speed with which enrollees qualified for Medicaid. If some were induced to enter assisted living earlier than they might have, they too may have used up funds that might have been available to support their own care over a longer period of time.

Disability policy research suggests that CLASS Act eligibility criteria, which many in the community could have met, would have induced some working disabled to leave the workforce. To ensure the fiscal soundness of the program, premiums for CLASS would have had to rise if steps were not taken to make it a less inviting insurance option for the already disabled and more inviting for the not-yet disabled. The requisite changes began to appear overwhelming, especially given the makeup of the current Congress. There now seems virtually no chance that Congress will, in the foreseeable future, move to the agenda a program to address the true catastrophic risk of long-term care, namely, nursing home care. This is especially true now that Congress has seen how difficult it is to address the selection and financing challenges so ineptly flirted with in the CLASS Act. Clearly, there is a market for long-term care insurance to cover what's called the continuum of long-term care: home visits, adult day care, respite care, meals on wheels, congregate feeding, transportation, alarm services, assisted living, and other supports. Of those who hold comprehensive long-term care insurance policies, research shows that the majority use their benefits to pay for home care and assisted living in about equal proportions, but 14% choose a nursing facility (Doty et al., 2010). For seniors who need nursing facility care and don't have insurance, especially for long stays, the CLASS Act would have brought little improvement to their lives. Its passage and subsequent quiet interment have made prospects for help even dimmer. What an odd memorial to Senator Ted Kennedy (D-MA), health care champion and advocate of publically subsidized long-term care services, in whose honor the legislation was passed with major input from his staff.

REFERENCES

AARP. (2006). *The costs of long-term care: Public perceptions versus reality in 2006.* Washington, DC: AARP.

Administration on Aging. (2010). *A profile of older Americans: 2010.* Washington, DC: Administration on Aging.

American Academy of Actuaries. (2009). *Letter to the U.S. Senate Committee on Health, Education, Labor and Pensions.* Retrieved from http://www.actuary.org/pdf/health/class_july09.pdf

America's Health Insurance Plans. (2007). *Long-term care insurance partnerships: New choices for consumers–potential savings for federal and state government.* Washington, DC: America's Health Insurance Plans.

Autor, D., & Duggan, M. (2003). The rise in disability rolls and the decline in unemployment. *Quarterly Journal of Economics, 118*(1), 157–205.

Burkhauser, R., & Daly, M. C. (2002). U.S. disability policy in a changing environment. *Journal of Economic Perspectives, 13*(2), 213–224.

Burkhauser, R., Houtenville, A. J., &Wittenburg, D. C. (2001). *A user guide to current statistics on the employment of people with disabilities.* Paper presented at the Conference on "The Persistence of Low Employment Rates of People With Disabilities—Cause and Policy Implications," October 18–19, Washington, DC. Retrieved from http://www.ilr.cornell.edu/ped/dep/files/Sec2/3_Burkhauser_Houtenville_Wittenburg.pdf

Castle, N. G., & Ferguson, J. C. (2011). What is nursing home quality and how is it measured? *The Gerontologist, 50*(4), 426–442.

Castle, N. G., Wagner, L. M., Ferguson, J. C., & Handler, S. M. (2011). Nursing home deficiency citations for safety. *Journal of Aging & Social Policy, 23*(1), 34–57.

Consumer Reports. (2006). Nursing homes: Business as usual. *Consumer Reports*. Retrieved from http://www.commonwealthfund.org/~/media/Files/Resources/2006/Nursing%20Homes%20%20A%20Consumer%20Reports%20Investigation/Sept06_Nursing_Homes%20pdf.pdf

Coughlin, T., Timothy, A., McBride, D., & Liu, K. (1990). Determinants of transitory and permanent nursing home admissions. *Medical Care, 28*(7), 616–631.

Doty, P. (2010). The evolving balance of formal and informal, institutional and non-institutional long-term care for older Americans: A thirty-year perspective. *Public Policy & Aging Report, 20*(1), 3–9.

Doty, P., Cohen, M. A., Miller, J., & Shi, X. (2010). Private long-term care insurance: Value to claimants and implication for long-term care financing. *The Gerontologist, 50*(5), 613–622.

Elder Guru. (n.d.). *CLASS Act long-term care insurance in the healthcare reform bill–good idea or bad?* Retrieved from http://www.elderguru.com/long-term-care-insurance-in-the-healthcare-reform-bill-good-idea-or-bad

Elmendorf, D. W. (2009). *Letter to honorable George Miller*. Washington, DC: Congressional Budget Office.

Elphinstone, J. W. (2010). Home prices drop despite ultra-low mortgage rates: Case-Shiller index. *The Huffington Post*. Retrieved from http://www.huffingtonpost.com/2010/05/25/case-shiller-march-2010-h_n_588501.html

Employee Benefits Research Institute. (2010). *Funding savings needed for health expenses for persons eligible for Medicare*. EBRI Issue Brief #351. Retrieved from http://www.ebri.org/pdf/briefspdf/EBRI_IB_12-2010_No351_Savings.pdf

Foster, R. S. (2009). *Updated and extended national health expenditure projections, 2010–2019*. Centers for Medicare & Medicaid Services. Retrieved from www.cms.gov/NationalHealthExpendData/downloads/NHE_Extended_Projections.pdf

Friedman, S. M., Steinwachs, D. M, Rathouz, P. J., Burton, L. C., & Mukamel, D. B. (2005). Characteristics predicting nursing home admission in the program of all-inclusive care for elderly people. *The Gerontologist, 45*(2), 157–166.

Gaugler, J. E, Duval, S., Anderson, K. A., & Kane, R. L. (2007). Predicting nursing home admission in the U.S.: A meta-analysis. *BMC Geriatrics, 7*, 13. Retrieved from http://www.biomedcentral.com/content/pdf/1471-2318-7-13.pdf

Genworth Life Insurance Company. (2010). *Beyond dollars, the true impact of long term caring*. Retrieved from http://www.ltc-associates.com/Docs/Beyond%20Dollars%20FINAL%20109048_093010_secure2011.pdf

Genworth Life Insurance Company. (2011). *Genworth 2011 cost of care Survey*. Retrieved from http://www.genworth.com/content/etc/medialib/genworth_v2/pdf/ltc_cost_of_care.Par.14625.File.dat/2010_Cost_of_Care_Survey_Full_Report.pdf

Grabowski, D. (2006). The cost-effectiveness of noninstitutional long-term care services: review and synthesis of the most recent evidence. *Medical Care Research and Review, 63*(1), 3–28.

Harrington, C. (2002). *Nursing home quality: State agency survey funding and performance*. Kaiser Family Foundation. Retrieved from http://www.kff.org/medicaid/loader.cfm?url=/commonspot/security/getfile.cfm&PageID=14105

Helman, R., Copeland C., & VanDerhei, J. (2010). *The 2010 Retirement Confidence Survey: Confidence stabilizing, but preparations continue to erode*. EBRI Issue

Brief, No. 340. Washington, DC. Retrieved from www.ebri.org/surveys/rcs/ 2010/

Kaiser Family Foundation. (n.d.). *Summary of the new health reform law.* Retrieved from www.kff.org/healthreform/upload/8061.pdf

Kaiser Family Foundation. (2007). *Views about the quality of long-term care services in the United States. 2007.* Retrieved from http://www.kff.org/kaiserpolls/upload/7718.pdf

Katz, S. (1972). *Effects of continued care: A study of chronic illness in the home.* Rockville, MD: National Center for Health Services Research and Development, DHEW publication No. (HSM) 73–3010.

Kemper, P., Applebaum, R., & Harrigan, M. (1987). Community care demonstrations: What have we learned? *Health Care Financing Review, 8*(4), 87–100.

Kingdon, J. (1995). *Agendas, alternatives and public policy* (2nd ed.). Glenview, IL: Addison-Wesley Educational Publishers, Inc.

Koff, S. (2010). Government to offer long-term-care insurance: Health care fact check. *The Cleveland Plain Dealer.* Retrieved from http://www.cleveland.com/medical/index.ssf/2010/04/health_care_fact_check_governm.html

Liu, K., Coughlin, T., & McBride, T. (1991). Predicting nursing-home admission and length of stay: A duration analysis. *Medical Care, 29*(2), 125–141.

Long-Term Care Insurance Tree (n.d.). *What are the chances of needing long term care?* Retrieved from http://www.longtermcareinsurancetree.com/ltc-basics/the-chances-of-needing-long-term-care.html

Meiners, M. (2011). *Connecting the long-term care partnership and CLASS Act insurance programs.* Retrieved from http://www.chcs.org/usr_doc/Partnership_Lessons_for_CLASS_-_FINAL.pdf

Mendes, E. (2010). *Lack of retirement funds is Americans' biggest financial worry.* Retrieved from http://www.gallup.com/poll/148058/Lack-Retirement-Funds-Americans-Biggest-Financial-Worry.aspx?utm_source=tagrss&utm_medium=rss&utm_campaign=syndication&utm_term=Well-Being Index

MetLife Mature Market Institute. (1999). *Metlife Juggling Act Study: Balancing caregiving with work and the costs involved.* Retrieved from http://www.caregiving.org/data/jugglingstudy.pdf

MetLife Mature Market Institute. (2011). *Caregiving costs to working caregivers.* Retrieved from http://www.guardianship.org/reports/mmi_caregiving_costs_working_caregivers.pdf

Miller, E. A., & Weissert, W. G. (2000). Predicting elderly people's risk for nursing home placement, hospitalization, functional impairment, and mortality. *Medical Care Research & Review, 57*(3), 259–297.

Miller E. A., Mor, V., & Clark, M. (2010). Reforming long-term care in the United States: Findings from a national survey of specialists. *The Gerontologist, 5*(2), 248–252.

Miller, E. A. (2011). Flying beneath the radar of health reform: The Community Living Assistance Services and Supports (CLASS) Act. *The Gerontologist, 51*(2), 145–155.

Moeller, P. (2009). Don't ignore likelihood of long-term care. *US News.* Retrieved from http://money.usnews.com/money/blogs/the-best-life/2009/10/01/dont-ignore-likelihood-of-long-term-care_print.html

Mor, V., Zinn, J., Angelelli, J., Teno, J. M., & Miller, S. C. (2004). Driven to tiers: Socioeconomic and racial disparities in the quality of nursing home care. *Milbank Quarterly*, *82*(2), 222–256.

Murtaugh, C. M., Kemper, P., Spillman, B. C., & Carlson, B. L. (1997). The amount, distribution, and timing of lifetime nursing home use. *Medical Care*, *35*(3), 204–218.

National Alliance for Caregiving. (2009). *Caregiving in the US 2009*. Retrieved from www.caregiving.org/data/Caregiving_in_the_US_2009_full_report.pdf

National Center for Health Statistics. (2002). *The National Nursing Home Survey: 1999 summary*. Washington, DC: U.S. Department of Health and Human Services. Retrieved from www.cdc.gov/nchs/data/nnhsd/Estimates/nnhs/Estimates_PaymentSource_Tables.pdf

Pauly, M. V. (1990). The rational nonpurchase of long-term-care insurance. *The Journal of Political Economy*, *98*(1), 153–168.

Pear, R. (2011). Long-term care needs changes, officials say. *The New York Times*. Retrieved from http://www.nytimes.com/2011/02/22/health/policy/22care.html?_r=1&sq=sebelius&st=cse

Pickert, K. (2009). Should long-term-care insurance be part of health reform? *Time*. Retrieved from http://www.time.com/time/politics/article/0,8599,1946431,00.html

Russell, D. W., Cutrona, C. E., de la Mora, A. & Wallace, R. B. (1997). Loneliness and nursing home admission among rural older adults. *Psychology and Aging*, *12*(4), 574–589.

Shesgreen, D. (2011). Federal officials wrestle with long-term insurance under health reform. *The Connecticut Mirror*. Retrieved from http://www.ctmirror.org

Spillman, B. C., Murtaugh, C. M., & Warshawsky, M. J. (2003). Policy implications of an annuity approach for integrating long-term care financing and retirement income. *Journal of Aging and Health*, *15*, 45–73.

The Federal Long-Term Care Insurance Program. (n.d.). *FLTCIP premium calculator*. Retrieved from https://www.ltcfeds.com/ltcWeb/do/assessing_your_needs/ratecalcOut

United States Central Intelligence Agency. (2010). *The world factbook* (online, updated biweekly, 2010 data). Retrieved from https://www.cia.gov/library/publications/the-world-factbook/rankorder/2004rank.html

U.S. Government Accountability Office. (2006). *Long-term care insurance: Federal program compared favorably with other products, and analysis of claims trend could inform future decisions*. GAO-06-401. Washington, DC.

Wiener, J. (2010). What does health reform mean for long-term care? *Public Policy and Aging Report*, *20*(2), 8.

Weissert, W. G., & Hedrick, S. C. (1994). Lessons learned from research on effects of community-based long-term care. *Journal of the American Geriatric Society*, *42*(3), 348–353.

Weissert, W. G., Cready, C, & Pawelak, J. (1988). The past and future of home and community-based long-term care. *The Milbank Quarterly*, *66*(2), 309–388.

Partnership Long-Term Care Insurance: Lessons for CLASS Program Development

MARK R. MEINERS, PhD

Professor of Health Administration and Policy, George Mason University, Fairfax, Virginia, USA

The Community Living Assistance Services and Supports (CLASS) Act was a voluntary public insurance strategy intended to help people pay for long-term care. CLASS was passed as part of health reform to overcome aspects of private long-term care insurance market failure but came under close scrutiny from both its supporters and its detractors. Experience with the long-term care insurance market and State Partnership Programs provide insights about how to make CLASS fiscally viable. A CLASS program that offered one set of options to cover front-end risk (e.g., 1 to 3 years) and another set to cover catastrophic risk (after a high deductible) could have been offered as an alternative to the basic CLASS "long and lean" benefit model with all enrollees joined into a single risk pool. This would have broadened the risk pool and lowered premium costs under the program.

INTRODUCTION

The Community Living Assistance Services and Supports (CLASS) provisions included in the Patient Protection and Affordable Care Act (ACA) establish a publically sponsored, voluntary long-term care insurance (LTCI) option for all working adults (Miller, 2011). In many ways this is a remarkable accomplishment (Manard, 2010). The ideas underlying CLASS had been around for many years without getting much traction. A cash program that was available to anyone, including those already disabled, was not seen as workable to private insurers. Nonetheless, the late Senator Kennedy and his staff successfully pushed to have CLASS included in the ACA, leaving many key details to be determined by the Department of Health and Human Services (DHHS) Secretary.

Within a year of its passage, DHHS Secretary Kathleen Sebelius (the Obama Administration official responsible for implementation of CLASS) announced the CLASS program was not sustainable without significant repairs (Sebelius, 2011). Technical adjustments suggested by Secretary Sebelius included increasing the work requirements to make it more difficult for those with disabilities to enroll, introducing an increasing premium structure to deal with inflation, tightening enrollment rules, and providing assistance and incentives for employers to participate. There was also one wild card suggestion in the mix that seemed especially conducive to opening the door to new options. The CLASS law said that the DHHS secretary was to be presented three alternatives from which one would be chosen as the CLASS plan made available to potential subscribers. But Secretary Sebelius said " . . . we're looking at ways to make the program appealing for Americans with a wide range of long-term care needs. A CLASS program that does not take a 'one-size-fits-all' approach will not only serve people better, it will also be attractive to larger number of people" (Sebelius, 2011).

Secretary Sebelius did not elaborate on what she had in mind, but experience from the current private market was under consideration as a point of reference. The CLASS office had hired an actuary with considerable expertise in private market LTCI to work out the challenges in the CLASS design. However, by late fall of 2011, the CLASS program development office was closed and a report was issued by the DHHS secretary that indicated the administration could not solve the many design problems posed by the CLASS legislation. The details of the final report suggest the problem may have had as much to do with the legal basis for undertaking technical corrections as with the actuarial challenges themselves (DHHS, 2011).

Although the CLASS Act has not been repealed, congressional support for technical corrections is not likely at this time. Still, there are many who hold out hope that deliberations involving CLASS can be revived once the current political climate is resolved. There also may be lessons learned from the work done to implement CLASS that would be useful in finding affordable and sustainable long-term care options. In this paper, that possibility is explored by comparing CLASS to private LTCI with special reference to the state-based LTCI Partnership Programs developed in 40 states across the country.

CLASS VERSUS PRIVATE LTCI

The CLASS Act was able to become law in part because CLASS benefits would have been sufficiently different from what is favored in the private market that it was not seen as a threat. In contrast to the CLASS one-size-fits-all approach, private LTCI offers a wide variety of benefit choices in such things as daily benefit amount (e.g., $50–$300), waiting time for benefits to begin after disability sets in (e.g., 0–90 days), and length of coverage (e.g., 1 year to lifetime). The benefits selected can have a significant effect on the premium. Other key features of private LTCI compared to the CLASS Act are outlined in Table 1.

There have been vigorous debates about the relationship between CLASS and private LTCI at the major annual meetings of insurers and their agents (Yee & Schoonveld, 2011; Thau & Slome, 2011). Some private insurance producers have come to feel the publicity around CLASS will help focus public attention on the need for LTCI, giving the market a positive boost and helping reverse the recent decline in market growth. Others feel at least as strongly that CLASS was a poorly constructed public program destined to need a taxpayer bailout (Blase & Hoff, 2011). Those concerns have fueled calls for the repeal of CLASS by the President's National Commission on Fiscal Responsibility and Reform (2010) and more recently contributed to the program being put on hold until further notice. It also was not clear that the DHHS secretary had the necessary flexibility to introduce creative options within the CLASS legislation (Congressional Research Service, 2011).

Underlying these hopes and fears are opposing political positions. Many advocates for CLASS do not like or trust private insurance. Many private

TABLE 1 Key Features of Long-Term Care Insurance and the CLASS Act

Program Features	LTC Insurance	CLASS
Underwriting of Risk	Yes	No
Regulation	States	Secretary of DHHS
Enrollment	Voluntary	Compulsory with voluntary opt-out option if offered by employer; voluntary otherwise
Employment Status	Not considered	Only for individuals who meet minimal earnings requirements
Waiting Period	Averages 90 days after you qualify to draw benefits	5-year waiting period before policies can be used, then must qualify to draw benefits
Legal Basis	Contracts enforceable by law	Federal entitlement program
Reserve Requirements	Collects premium and invests in reserves	Reserves are treasury bonds

insurance advocates see public options as unwanted alternatives that "crowd out" the private market (Moses, 2005).

Everyone on all sides of the issue acknowledges that the LTCI market is underdeveloped relative to its potential and certainly relative to the need for such protection.

An important goal of CLASS was to expand on what private LTCI has accomplished in getting people financially prepared for the risk of needing long term services and supports. When LTCI policies first emerged in the 1980s, they were mostly nursing home–only policies, but today an estimated 92% have comprehensive coverage for both institutional and noninstitutional care, including custodial home- and community-based services (HCBS) as well as care in assisted living (Cohen, 2011). By 2010, typical benefits chosen averaged $154 per day and can be used to reimburse costs for a wide range of long term services and supports, usually going into effect following a 90-day waiting period. Eligibility for benefits is typically established once a beneficiary has at least two to three limitations in activities of daily living that are expected to last at least 90 days or when a beneficiary is cognitively impaired and requires ongoing supervision. The benefit duration sold has been relatively constant over the past 15 years, averaging around 5 years (Cohen, 2011).

With private LTCI, there has been considerable controversy surrounding whether, how, and how much to adjust for inflation. In the early years of LTCI, it was typical to sell coverage with little or no inflation protection. More recently, buyers have begun to be educated that having good inflation protection is a key indicator of the quality of the coverage. Without adequate inflation protection, the proportion of care covered decreases over time to the point that it may leave the beneficiary with larger than expected gaps in coverage.

In 2010, 95% of new sales had some form of inflation protection (American Association for Long-Term Care Insurance, 2011). Still, it is easy to get confused by the many different kinds of inflation adjustments that have been introduced. Whether the inflation rate is designed to increase on a compound basis (each increase builds on the previous increase) or simple basis (each increase is a set amount of the base premium) and whether it is to be 5%, 3%, or the consumer price index, all will affect the level of premium charged, which in turn affects sales.

A recent update on the LTCI market indicated about 8 million policies in force with about 70% of them sold in the individual market (Cohen, 2011). But annual individual sales have been declining or flat since 2002, and a number of companies have exited the market due to the low interest rate earnings on reserves and a poor sales experience in a tough economy. The group market has been growing somewhat relative to the individual market, but overall market penetration is small, estimated at between 3% and

6% depending on assumptions about potential buyers (Cutler, Spillman, & Tell, 2010).

CLASS intended to overcome some of the perceived areas of market failure by offering a very different approach from the private market. The most notable and challenging feature was that working disabled people and others who might be excluded by private insurance underwriting could be covered by CLASS. That is, there was to be no underwriting of the risk. CLASS also went further than private insurance by offering subsidized coverage for full-time students younger than 22 and working individuals who have incomes below the poverty level but not eligible for Medicaid. These individuals were to pay a modest premium of $5 per month, adjusted by the Consumer Price Index in urban areas (CPI-U). These reduced premiums would have been subsidized by higher premiums paid by the broader risk pool of CLASS participants. The CLASS legislation explicitly excluded drawing from the general federal treasury to pay for any aspect of the program.

The basic CLASS benefit design was different from the typical private product outlined above. Once a beneficiary became eligible, a cash payment was to be made available for as long as the beneficiary needed it. The legislation specified an average daily benefit of no less than $50 daily (indexed for inflation) but allowed it to vary based on the degree of disability or impairment. The CLASS authors envisioned that a low daily benefit approach would help to keep the premium low and allow for private market supplementation. Beneficiaries would have an amount available that when combined with Social Security would be used to buy basic services and supports that helped them age in place without having to go to nursing homes. If they needed nursing home care, they could use it there, but the design favored HCBS.

Indeed, the amounts paid out were not intended to cover the full cost of care, especially at the nursing home level of dependency. In 2011, the national median cost for a semiprivate room in a nursing home was $193 per day; for assisted living it was $109 per day; and for licensed home health aide services it was $19 an hour (Genworth, 2011). If that cash payment was not enough to keep someone from spending down and becoming Medicaid-eligible, CLASS benefits were to be supplemented by Medicaid payments for Medicaid-covered services. CLASS enrollees who received HCBS would have been allowed to retain 50% of the CLASS benefit, the other half being used to offset Medicaid's costs. For institutional care, Medicaid would have received 95% of the CLASS payment, with the beneficiary keeping the remaining 5%.

In contrast, private LTCI provides no subsidies for students, for those with low income, or those eligible for Medicaid. Alternatively, about 30% to 40% of private LTCI premiums are used for administrative and marketing expenses along with profit. With CLASS, only 3% of the premium would have been allowed for administration and marketing. CLASS designers had looked to employers as keys to marketing the program. Employers who offered the CLASS program would enroll all their employees, who could then choose to opt out. Most analysts saw big challenges with this given other demands of health reform on employers. Even with the visibility of a government-run program, overhead costs would more likely still have needed to be in the 15% to 20% range for CLASS. Private LTCI experience over many years has found that the public does not understand the financial risk, much less how to prepare for it. The small overhead allowance for marketing was one of the many concerns that worried the CLASS office (DHHS, 2011).

CONTROLLING CLASS RISKS

Although it would not have engaged in underwriting, the CLASS program would have included some eligibility restrictions to help reduce adverse selection (overrepresentation of bad risks in the insured population). The program would have been limited to working adults 18 years or older. Retirees and non-working people with disabilities would not have been eligible to enroll. In addition, there was to be a 5-year waiting period during which enrollees would have had to pay premiums before they could make claims. In at least 3 of those years, they would have had to have employment paying an amount at least equal to one-quarter of Social Security coverage (i.e., $1,120 in 2011). These restrictions were intended to demonstrate that CLASS was not intended for those who already require constant long-term care.

Among the adjustments considered was further tightening the eligibility rules. The Joint Academy/Society of Actuaries CLASS Act Task Force had called for a substantial increase in the work requirement, a minimum of 20 to 30 hours of scheduled work per week or a comparable requirement (Schmitz, 2011). The Academy of Actuaries also called for restrictions on the ability to opt out and subsequently opt back in. The CLASS office considered requiring a full 5 years of employment instead of just 3 years and increasing the annual earnings to $12,000, the amount required by the Social Security Administration for a non-blind person to be engaged in "substantially gainful activity" (DHHS, 2011).

SUPPLEMENT TO LTCI MARKET

The limited cash benefit of CLASS along with the flexibility of private LTCI invited the possibility for private wraparound products to fill gaps in the CLASS benefit. The feasibility of a private supplemental market emerging to fill gaps in CLASS coverage would have largely depended on the affordability of CLASS. Most individuals seeking LTCI can likely afford only one policy. However, if the cost of CLASS were low enough and the value was appealing to those interested in LTCI, then a supplemental market could arise. France, a distant second in private LTCI sales to the United States, has a compulsory public insurance program that pays small cash benefits relative to the cost of care (Taleyson, 2003). Since the payment also decreases with income, the program has been credited with prompting the rapid growth of private "wraparound" insurance as a complement to the compulsory public benefit, particularly among the financially better off (Gleckman, 2010; Ludden, 2009).

MULTIPLE CLASS OPTIONS

The CLASS office also introduced the idea of a family of options. This would have allowed for the possibility of pooling the risk so there could be cross-subsidization among the options made available. The idea of a family of plan choices made sense for several reasons. Selling only one basic option is likely to limit the market more than is optimal. There is no unique level that defines catastrophic long-term care–related expenditures; it can vary for each individual. The low cash benefit for a lifetime "long and lean" approach is not likely to provide catastrophic protection for anyone, so other options should be considered. Although the idea of a limited cash benefit, as envisioned in CLASS, seemed appealing as a way to hold down costs, focus groups run by the CLASS office specifically mentioned they preferred a benefit that covered more of the total cost of long-term care (DHHS, 2011). More options could have broadened the risk pool and helped spread the overhead costs.

It would have been helpful if those developing alternatives to the basic CLASS model gave fuller consideration to the German experience with a limited cash benefit. CLASS was inspired in part by the popularity of the German social LTCI program. Germany offers beneficiaries a choice between having their long-term care services paid for through an agency-directed service-denominated benefit or to receive a consumer-directed cash benefit. Although valued at just 20% to 53% of the agency-directed benefit, depending on category of need, the cash option was initially a very popular choice; 83% of eligible Germans choose to self-direct their benefits in 1995 (Karlsson, 2002). However, more recently, when given this choice, Germans have shown greater preference for agency services with most people not choosing to oversee their own care (von Schwanenflugel, 2011). In part this may be because the cash payment does not cover the full bill when people need high levels of care like those provided in nursing homes and assisted living facilities.

In the United States, some private LTCI policies offer cash benefits, but most do not. Cash benefits are viewed by most private insurers as easier to use and harder to administer than service reimbursed benefits, so the premiums average as much as 40% higher to compensate for the greater risk of induced demand and moral hazard. The cash benefit in CLASS had strong support from disability advocates and others favoring consumer-directed care (Miller, 2011). But in the context of a family of CLASS plan options, perhaps the choice of reimbursement-only benefits like those in the private LTCI market could have been considered as a way to lower costs.

CLASS BENEFIT LIMITATIONS

Another possible option to consider for lowering premiums is to limit the benefit to something other than lifetime. Lifetime protection has become a less popular focus for private LTCI sales agents because premiums had to be raised to adjust for higher than expected payouts due to fewer people dropping their insurance and lower earnings on reserves because of declining interest rates. There is also a growing recognition that lifetime coverage gives no incentive to budget the available benefit once a beneficiary becomes eligible for payments.

Among the adjustments the CLASS office did consider was to use a 15-year exclusion period during which no payments would be made if the claim involved a preexisting medical condition knowable at the time of enrollment. Another was to have the daily benefit amount increase with the level of impairment in the first 5 years of use but then cutting the amount substantially after that. Another had the daily benefit increasing the longer the CLASS policy was held without going into claim, rising from $20 per day after the vesting period to $150 per day after 25 years, with the payout limited to 3 years. The level of complexity in the changes necessary to put CLASS on firmer financial footing contributed to the abandonment of the CLASS program (DHHS, 2011).

CLASS INFLATION PROTECTION INNOVATION

One of the more innovative adjustments considered by the CLASS office was to differentiate how CLASS would provide inflation protection compared to what is typically done with private LTCI. The CLASS legislation required the benefit to be indexed for inflation as measured by the CPI-U, but it was silent on how to build the inflation adjustment into premiums. The approach suggested by the CLASS actuary was to build inflation protection into the premiums over time by the same rate CPI-U used to increase the benefits. This "flexible increasing premium option" idea has also been proposed for private market offerings, but has not yet been generally adopted (Soppe, Yee, & Markusfeld, 2007).

While the need to adjust benefits for inflation may seem obvious, it can be quite complicated. Before elaborating further on this point, I digress briefly to point out that with or without inflation protection, premiums in private LTCI are typically designed to be level over the life of the premium, and CLASS was to follow this approach. As people age, their risk of needing long-term care goes up, which means the starting premium will be higher the longer one waits to buy insurance. If starting premiums are then also "age-adjusted" after purchase, they would increase over time as people age. Level premiums, rather than age-adjusted premiums, have been the private LTCI norm because they encourage consumers to prefund the risk prior to retirement. This helps consumers avoid letting their policies "lapse" at older ages when benefits are most needed, but it also means that the starting premium is higher than if it were to be age-adjusted.

To understand the significance of what the CLASS actuarial team proposed, it is important to understand that including inflation protection in a level premium structure can result in significantly higher premiums, and the effect can be dramatic depending on the age the insurance is first purchased. Consider, for example, the premiums calculated under various assumptions for policies sold in the recent federal LTCI program (Federal Long-Term Care Insurance Program Premium Calculation, 2011). A lifetime policy paying $100 per day after a 90-day deductible period, without inflation protection built into the premium, costs $28 per month if purchased at age 45, $52 per month if purchased at age 55, and $102 per month if purchased at age 65. These premiums are designed to stay level over the life of the policy. The same baseline policy with an annual 5% compound inflation factor built into the level premium would cost $119 if purchased at age 45, $174 per month if purchased at age 55, and $267 per month if purchased at age 65. In other words, at age 45, the starting premium is more than four times higher if inflation is built into a level premium structure. At age 65, the level premium is still more than two and half times higher if inflation is built into a level premium structure. The approach proposed by the CLASS actuarial would have built in the inflation adjustment over time so that premiums would increase gradually with the general cost of living, making CLASS much more affordable at younger ages.

STATE LTCI PARTNERSHIP PROGRAMS

Private insurers and states have joined together in establishing LTCI Partnership Programs that share with CLASS the public policy goal of helping middle-class consumers prepare for the risk of catastrophic long-term care costs. Both the CLASS and Partnership Programs are designed to address issues in LTCI that have limited the reach of the private market (Meiners, 2011). The Partnership LTCI strategy, operating so far in 40 states, is built directly on private LTCI products currently offered in the market place. By December 2010, the combination of new and old partnership states had some 540,000 Partnership policies in force (Long-Term Care Partnership Program, 2011a, 2011b). In what follows, considerations underlying the Partnership strategy are offered that suggest options for CLASS that had the potential to increase significantly the number of people who would have participated in CLASS and purchased LTCI more generally.

Partnership programs were launched in the early 1990s. At that time, the newly emerging market for private LTCI was focused primarily on purchasers in the upper end of the income and asset spectrum. A few states (California, Connecticut, Indiana, and New York), with support from the Robert Wood Johnson Foundation (RWJF), worked to broaden the market to middle-income consumers most at risk of depleting their limited resources and needing Medicaid assistance. These states promoted the purchase of private LTCI by offering special Medicaid eligibility rules that allow enhanced asset protection if additional long-term care coverage was needed beyond what a person's policy provides (Meiners, McKay, & Mahoney, 2002).

The Partnership incentive strategy served as the model for the National Partnership Program passed by Congress with the 2005 Deficit Reduction Act, which allowed the program to expand beyond the four original states (RWJF, 2007). While the core features are essentially the same for Partnership and non-Partnership LTCI policies, one key distinction is that private LTCI providers have to follow certain rules regarding inflation protection to qualify as Partnership products (Meiners, 2007). Compound inflation protection is required for purchasers aged 60 or younger, simple (no compounding) inflation adjustments are required for purchasers who are age 61 to 75, and purchasers aged 76 or older can forgo inflation protection. In states that have adopted the program, insurance companies can voluntarily agree to participate by offering LTCI coverage that meets state and federal requirements for inflation protection along with requirements on agent training and reporting on policies sold.

As with the original four state programs, the expanded Partnership Program incentivizes take-up by allowing consumers to avoid being impoverished if they need help from Medicaid (Meiners, 2008). If a person's long-term care needs exceed their coverage, they are permitted to keep assets up to the amount that the insurance plan has paid and still get help from Medicaid (i.e., a dollar of extra asset protection under Medicaid rules for every dollar LTCI pays out). For example, a policy could pay out $60,000, and if the covered individual needed more care but had exhausted his or her coverage and/or spent assets down to $60,000, the special "asset disregard" provisions offered by Partnership states allow them to keep $60,000 and still receive extended care through Medicaid. Otherwise, the person would have had to spend all but about $2,000 of savings before Medicaid could help. On average, people who use formal long-term care use it for 3 years or less, so front-end protection is especially helpful (Murtaugh, Kemper, & Spillman, 1997; Kemper, Komisar, & Alecxih, 2005/2006).

With Partnership as with private LTCI in general, the choice of how to limit the benefit is left to the purchaser, with a wide array of options that can be tailored to individual preferences and budgets. Waiting periods, daily copays, and other gaps in coverage will lower premiums, but these gaps must be self-insured so they should only be as large as can be easily handled out-of-pocket. Partnership insurance allows the biggest gap in coverage to be when the insurance no longer pays anything. This gap can vary by the total dollar amount/length of protection the person feels he or she can buy.

Partnership LTCI is especially intended to help insurable consumers from the "middle mass" market defined by a Society of Actuaries study on retirement to be the segment of the population representing 83% of households generally suited for purchasing a LTCI product (Society of Actuaries, 2010). The average household income of this group in the ages leading up to retirement (55 to 64) is estimated to be $75,000, with average assets net of home values at just over $100,000. Many in this group end up self-insuring (i.e., paying for services and supports out of pocket) even though it puts them at greater risk of impoverishment.

The Partnership strategy allows the purchaser to consider limits in coverage that can help make the premium affordable. Conversely, Partnership insurance results in Medicaid savings if most policy holders end up with insurance that pays more than they could have spent from their savings on long-term care before becoming Medicaid eligible. Several of the original RWJF Partnership states have estimated Medicaid savings from their programs (Meiners, 2009).

MULTIPLE CLASS OPTIONS RECONSIDERED IN LIGHT OF LTCI EXPERIENCE

The idea of having a family of options within CLASS could have opened up other policy designs that help with adverse selection along with other aspects of market failure that are not so obvious. By incorporating options that focus on limited segments of the risk, the provision of multiple CLASS options could have served to stimulate areas of the private LTCI market that have been undeveloped relative to what is needed.

The affordability of CLASS options would have been dependent on the size of the risk pool, which itself is dependent on the premium charged (Tumlinson, Ng, & Hammelman, 2010). Estimates ranged from as low as an average of $60 per month when mandatory enrollment is assumed to $240 per month when 2% of the population enrolls, and those averages were expected to vary by age (Manard, 2010). One estimate by the CLASS actuary went as high as $3,000 a month when extreme levels of adverse selection were assumed (DHHS, 2011). But if large numbers of individuals with "good" insurance risk were attracted to CLASS this could have reduced the effect of adverse selection and helped keep premiums competitive with private LTCI.

Since its inception, the Partnership Program has tried to encourage "short and fat" products that offered inflation-protected comprehensive benefits but for limited periods of time (preferably in the range of the dollar equivalent of 1 to 3 years of coverage) as a way to broaden sales to the middle mass market. The idea is that everyone could benefit from as little as a year or two of coverage when a long-term care crisis hits. Indeed, many in the middle mass market do not see themselves as being able to afford more than that. But the success of Partnership Programs has been limited by industry resistance to making "short and fat" products a priority. Agents are commission-driven to sell higher benefit amounts per policy, for example, 3 years or more. From 1990 to 2005, the average benefits duration of policies sold has been in the range of 5.5 years. The 2010 numbers indicate a decrease to 4.8 years, possibly due to the advent of the Partnership Program but more likely the result of a very weak economy (Cohen, 2011).

Some success has been demonstrated in long-standing Partnership states—policies covering the equivalent of 2 years or less comprise 26% of Partnership sales in California and 34% of Partnership sales in Connecticut. Sales of 3-year products have captured another 25% of the market in California and 33% in Connecticut. However, these examples are exceptions and only a beginning. On a national basis, only 8% of all individual private LTCI sales in 2010 covered less than 3 years; another 28% had a 3-year benefit period (American Association for Long-Term Care Insurance, 2011).

Although high-end sales are easier and more lucrative for agents, the bulk of the potential market is not high-end. Of those households viewed as suitable for LTCI products, only 17% comprise the "middle-affluent" segment where potential buyers' pre-retirement household incomes average $132,000 and net assets average $390,000 (Society of Actuaries, 2010). This segment is much more limited than the middle mass market, but there are still enough potential purchasers to hold the focus for the relatively few agents who specialize in LTCI.

Furthermore, the few sales made in the middle mass market still tend to be high-end products. In 2005, for example, the average benefit duration was 5.1 years for those with incomes of $25,000 to $49,000 and 5.3 years for those with incomes of $50,000 to $74,999, compared to 5.6 years for those with incomes of $75,000 or more (LifePlans, 2007). This has been a troubling form of market failure, especially if purchasers with lower incomes are giving up inflation protection to get the extended coverage that was a common trade off in the early years of the market.

Making 1- to 3-year equivalent products an option in the CLASS program could have served to stimulate this important segment of the market by attracting good risks that can only afford limited benefits. The choice can have a significant effect on the premium. For example, in the earlier example from the federal LTCI offering, a lifetime policy with a 90-day waiting period covering $100 per day, indexed for 5% annual compound inflation, costs a 55-year-old purchaser $174 per month. If the same person were to limit this coverage to 2 years, the policy would cost less than half this amount ($81 per month). If such a policy had Partnership asset protection, the beneficiary could access Medicaid support and retain as much as $73,000 ($100 × 365 days × 2 years) for other uses.

Options within CLASS at the other end of the benefit spectrum could have also helped with market failure that exists for those only interested in catastrophic protection. For many years, lifetime protection was a major focus of the LTCI industry. But lifetime benefits are only available when packaged with relatively short deductibles of 90 days or less, after which you could be covered as long as needed. This makes that coverage expensive, and people who only want true catastrophic-only protection may be put off by the high price.

A CLASS high-deductible catastrophic benefit design (e.g., 2- to 5-year deductible) would be attractive to buyers from along the wealth spectrum who are willing to self-insure large amounts of their long-term care expenses but want a stop-loss insurance policy to back them up. Using the premiums for the comprehensive federal LTCI policy example used earlier ($100 daily benefit with 5% compound inflation), the catastrophic lifetime benefit would be reduced from $173 per month to an estimated $93 per month if the deductible period was the equivalent of 2 years instead of 90 days; a 3-year deductible would drop the monthly premium estimate to $70, and a 5-year deductible would lower it to $48 per month. With catastrophic options, CLASS could have attracted better than average risks with significant resources that might otherwise self-insure. A catastrophic benefit structure like this would provide those purchasers with the peace of mind that their long-term care losses would be limited to an amount they could afford.

A CLASS program that offers options that cover the limited segments of the front-end risk (e.g., 1 to 3 years) and another set that covers the catastrophic risk after a high deductible could have been offered as alternative options to the basic CLASS model with all enrollees joined into a single risk pool. The new CLASS options would have been significantly less expensive than the original CLASS option. Because each option would be attractive to different market segments, the combined risk pool could have been much larger than if only the "long and lean" option had been offered.

IMPLICATIONS

One widely acknowledged benefit of CLASS is an increase in public awareness about the importance of insuring against long-term care risk. This factor seems to have been overlooked in the push to have CLASS repealed. The private insurance market needs a boost. Some prominent insurers have left the market recently, and the overall number has generally been in decline over recent years (Lieber, 2010). For those insurers who remain in the market, good risk selection is one of the keys to profitability, so the incentive for insurers that remain in the market is to err on the conservative side.

We know little about private market underwriting practices, but what we do know suggests that underwriting keeps the market smaller than what CLASS advocates are trying to achieve. Still, one study estimated that if everyone applied at age 65, between just 12% and 23% would be rejected (Murtaugh et al., 1995). This suggests there are far more insurable risks than insured people. On the other hand, another study estimated that at least one older person in seven who had been rejected may not represent more risk than those accepted (Temkin-Greener, Mukamel, & Meiners, 2001). This, too, suggests that there are more good risks than what the private market now covers. An array of front-end only and back-end only options offered along with the legislated CLASS benefit could attract a wider variety of risk preferences, increasing the risk pool and reducing adverse selection.

Another important benefit is that CLASS would have provided coverage for individuals who do not meet the underwriting requirements of private insurance. However, the basic CLASS benefit structure was not right for everyone, and the program clearly faced significant challenges associated with adverse selection. Allowing the DHHS secretary to consider options that cover limited segments at the front-end and back-end of the risk distribution could have helped lower premiums and attract a larger risk pool. These segments have been subject to market failure in the private market yet have potential appeal to insurable individuals who might be attracted to such coverage. Revising CLASS to include these additional options could have reduced program costs, through both the provision of cheaper options in addition to expansion of the risk pool.

If adding the proposed options to CLASS proved successful, private market policies would have emerged to challenge the new CLASS options, and competition would have ensued. This would serve the broader public policy goal by further reducing the price of such policies and helping to incentivize significantly more people to prepare financially for the risk of long-term care.

Thus, if technical modifications become possible for the CLASS program, allowing more CLASS options would be an important adjustment that could help address the potential for adverse selection problems while significantly increasing the number of people who have long-term care assistance either through CLASS or private LTCI.

More sales are needed in the middle-income market segment where people are most at risk for spending down their resources if basic levels of LTCI coverage are not in place. The front-end benefit strategy promoted by state Partnership Programs should be incorporated into a revived CLASS program to help meet the program's goal of making financial planning more affordable and appealing to those in the middle mass market.

Offering very high–deductible catastrophic options in CLASS could also help by drawing into the CLASS risk pool those who are willing to self-insure for as much as 2 to 5 years of care but want catastrophic-level coverage if more care is needed. An array of front-end only and back-end only options offered along with the legislated CLASS model would allow for lower cost options and attract a wider variety of risk preferences. This would increase the CLASS risk pool and reduce adverse selection.

REFERENCES

American Association for Long-Term Care Insurance. (2011). *LTCi Sourcebook.* Westlake Village, CA: Author.

Blase, B., & Hoff, J .S. (2011). *Secretary Sebelius cannot fix CLASS*. The Heritage Foundation, WebMemo, No. 3193, March 16.

Cohen, M. A. (2011). *Financing long-term care: The private insurance market.* Presented at National Health Policy Forum, Washington, DC, April 15.

Congressional Research Service. (2011). *Memorandum to Rep. Charles Boustany Jr.,* March 15.

Cutler, J. A., Spillman, B., & Tell, E. J. (2010). *Private financing of long term care: market penetration and market potential.* Presentation at Academy Health ARM Conference, Boston, MA, June.

Department of Health and Human Services (DHHS). (2011). *A report on the actuarial, marketing, and legal analysis of the CLASS Program.* Retrieved from http://aspe.hhs.gov/daltcp/reports/2011/class/index.shtml

Federal Long-Term Care Insurance Program Premium Calculation. (2011). Retrieved from https://www.ltcfeds.com/ltcWeb/do/assessing_your_needs/ratecalcOut

Genworth. (2010). *Cost of care survey.* Retrieved from http://www.genworth.com/content/products/long_term_care/long_term_care/cost_of_care.html

Gleckman, H. (2010). *Long-term care financing reform: Lessons from the U.S. and abroad.* New York, NY: The Commonwealth Fund.

Kemper, P., Komisar, H. L., & Alecxih, L. (2005/2006). long-term care over an uncertain future: What can current retirees expect? *Inquiry, 42,* 335–350.

Karlsson, M. (2002). *Comparative analysis of long-term care systems in four countries. international institute for applied systems analysis.* Interim Report IR-02-003, January. Retrieved from http://www.iiasa.ac.at/Admin/PUB/Documents/IR-02-003.pdf

Lieber, R. (2010). When a safety net is yanked away. *New York Times*, November 13. Retrieved from http://www.nytimes.com/2010/11/13/your-money/13money.html

LifePlans, Inc. (2007). *Who buys long-term care insurance? A 15-year study of buyers and non-buyers, 1990–2005.* America's Health Insurance Plans. Retrieved from http://www.ahipresearch.org/PDFs/LTC_Buyers_Guide.pdf

Long-Term Care Partnership Program. (2011a). *DRA Partnership reports*. Retrieved from http://w2.dehpg.net/LTCPartnership/Reports.aspx

Long-Term Care Partnership Program. (2011b). *Other Partnership reports*. Retrieved from http://w2.dehpg.net/LTCPartnership/generic.aspx?idir=other%20reports

Ludden, B. (2009). *View from abroad: LTC Insurance in Canada, Germany, France, and the UK*. Presentation at Ninth Annual Intercompany Long-Term Care Insurance Conference. Reno, NV: March 31.

Manard, B. (2010). Dueling talking points: Technical issues in constructing and passing the CLASS Act. *Public Policy and Aging Report*, *20*(2), 21–27.

Meiners, M. R., & McKay, H. L. (1990). Public vs. private insurance: Beware the comparison. *Generations*, *14*(2), 32–40.

Meiners, M. R., McKay, H. L., & Mahoney, K. J. (2002). Partnership insurance: An innovation to meet LTC financing needs in an era of Federal Minimalism. *Journal of Aging and Social Policy*, *14*(3/4), 75–83.

Meiners, M. R. (2007). *Long-term care partnership: State considerations for inflation protection*. Center for Health Care Strategies, Inc. Policy Brief, August.

Meiners, M. R. (2008). *Medicaid eligibility issues for long-term care Partnership Programs*. Center for Health Care Strategies, Inc. Policy Brief, March.

Meiners, M. R. (2009). *Long-term care insurance partnership: Considerations for cost-effectiveness*. Center for Health Care Strategies, Inc. Policy Brief, March.

Meiners, M. R. (2011). *Connecting the long-term care Partnership and CLASS Act insurance programs*. Center for Health Care Strategies, Inc. Policy Brief, February.

Miller, E. A. (2011). Flying beneath the radar of health reform: The Community Living Assistance Services and Supports (CLASS) Act. *The Gerontologist*, *51*(2), 145–155.

Moses, S. A. (2005). *Aging America's Achilles' heel: Medicaid long-term care*. Washington, DC: Cato Institute.

Murtaugh, C. M., Kemper P., & Spillman B. C. (1995). Risky business: Long-term care insurance underwriting. *Inquiry*, *32*(3), 271–284.

National Commission on Fiscal Responsibility and Reform. (2010). *The moment of truth. The White House*. Retrieved from http://www.fiscalcommission.gov/sites/fiscalcommission.gov/files/documents/TheMomentofTruth12_1_2010.pdf

Robert Wood Johnson Foundation. (2007). *Long-term care Partnership expansion: A new opportunity for states*. Issue Brief, May. Retrieved from http://www.chcs.org/usr_doc/Long-Term_Care_Partnership_Expansion.pdf

Sebelius, K. (2011). *Kaiser Family Foundation briefing on long-term care*. February 7. Retrieved from http://www.hhs.gov/secretary/about/speeches/sp20110207.html

Schmitz, A. (2011). Hearing on the implementation and sustainability of the new government-administered Community Living Assistance Services and Supports (CLASS) Program, Committee on Energy and Commerce Subcommittee on Health, United States House of Representatives, March 17.

Society of Actuaries. (2010, March 17). *Long-term care think tank report: LTCi: From hope to change*. Schaumberg, IL: Author.

Soppe, J., Yee, B., & Markusfeld, H. (2007). *A superior LTCi product design*. Senior Health Management Corporation presentation, July 30.

Taleyson, L. (2003). *Private LTC insurance: International comparisons.* SCOR technical Newsletters. Retrieved from http://www.actuaries.org/IAAHS/OnlineJournal/2006-1/scorltc1.pdf

Temkin-Greener, H., Mukamel, D. B., & Meiners, M. R. (2001). Long-term care insurance underwriting: Understanding eventual claims experience. *Inquiry, 37*(4), 348–358.

Thau, C., & Slome, J. (2011). *Selling in the presence of the CLASS Act.* Session LTC922. American Association for Long-Term Care Insurance 9th Long-Term Care Insurance Producers Summit, Las Vegas, NV.

Tumlinson, A., Ng, W., & Hammelman, E. (2010). The circular relationship between enrollment and premiums: Effects on the CLASS Program Act. *Public Policy and Aging Report, 20*(2), 28–30.

von Schwanenflugel, M. (2011). CLASS Act: Lessons for the long-term care challenges in America and Germany. *The Journal AARP International.* Summer.

Yee, R., & Schoonveld, S. (2011). *CLASS Act–Where is it at–Where is it going + experts answer your questions.* Session LTC919. American Association for Long-Term Care Insurance 9th Long-Term Care Insurance Producers Summit, Las Vegas, NV.

Medicaid Home- and Community-Based Services: Impact of the Affordable Care Act

CHARLENE HARRINGTON, PhD

Professor, Department of Social and Behavioral Sciences, University of California, San Francisco, San Francisco, California, USA

TERENCE NG, JD, MA

Senior Research Analyst, Department of Social and Behavioral Sciences, University of California, San Francisco, San Francisco, California, USA

MITCHELL LaPLANTE, PhD and H. STEPHEN KAYE, PhD

Professors, Institute for Health and Aging, University of California, San Francisco, San Francisco, California, USA

The Affordable care Act (ACA) legislation of 2010 has three important voluntary provisions for the expansion of home- and community-based services (HCBS) under Medicaid: A state can choose to (1) offer a community first choice option to provide attendant care services and supports; (2) amend its state plan to provide an optional HCBS benefit; and (3) rebalance its spending on long term services and supports to increase the proportion that is community-based. The first and third provisions offer states enhanced federal matching rates as an incentive. Although the new provisions are valuable, the law does not set minimum standards for access to HCBS, and the new financial incentives are limited especially for the many states facing serious budget problems. Wide variations in access to HCBS can be expected to continue, while HCBS will continue to compete for funding with mandated institutional services.

INTRODUCTION

State Medicaid programs are jointly funded by the federal and state governments. At 42% of total U.S. long-term care (LTC) expenditures, Medicaid plays a major role for individuals who meet state financial eligibility and needs-based criteria to qualify for Medicaid payment of these services (Hartman, Martin, McDonnell, Catlin, & National Health Expenditure Accounts Team, 2009). As the costs of LTC services have increased over time, Medicaid has become a critical resource for low-income individuals with disabilities.

When the Medicaid program was established, nursing home services and home health were mandatory benefits, but other home- and community-based services (HCBS) were optional. As a result, institutional services grew rapidly and HCBS were slow to develop. The federal government has since established the HCBS waiver program and state plan optional benefit programs and have greatly expanded HCBS through a number of initiatives. These efforts have been encouraged by the growing demand of individuals who want HCBS and their advocates' involvement in the policy arena (Kitchener, Ng, Miller, & Harrington, 2005). The 1999 U.S. Supreme Court ruling in *Olmstead v. L.C.* found that unnecessary institutionalization of individuals is a type of discrimination prohibited by the Americans with Disabilities Act (Carlson & Coffey, 2010). Since then, a number of Olmstead legal actions have challenged the limited state access to Medicaid HCBS and have encouraged states to expand their programs.

The primary focus of this paper is to review the major provisions for the expansion of Medicaid HCBS in the Affordable Care Act (ACA), signed into law by President Obama in March 2010. For background, this paper will describe current state Medicaid HCBS programs, some recent initiatives to expand access to these services, and barriers to care. Finally, we will analyze the potential impact of the ACA provisions and identify some of the current problems not addressed by the ACA.

BACKGROUND

Trends in HCBS Programs

The three major state Medicaid HCBS programs are (1) HCBS waivers, (2) home health, and (3) personal care services. The HCBS waiver program (under Section 1915(c) of the Social Security Act) allows states to waive

Medicaid requirements to target specific population groups. States can provide services otherwise not covered by the state Medicaid plan, but they are allowed to limit services to specific population groups and geographical areas and to limit the total number of participants served (Kitchener et al., 2005). HCBS waivers are limited to individuals who meet the state eligibility requirements for institutional care, and aggregate program costs cannot be more expensive than institutional services for an equivalent population (i.e., they must be cost-neutral). The HCBS waivers typically offer many services such as case management and personal care. The home health benefit usually requires the need for professional services such as nursing or therapy and may provide home health aide services. Home health services must be offered on a statewide basis to all age and population groups who meet the state need criteria. Personal care services under the state plan option, offered by 32 states, provide basic assistance with activities of daily living, and they also must be offered on a statewide basis to all age and population groups who meet the state need criteria (Kitchener et al., 2005; Kitchener, Ng, & Harrington, 2007; Ng, Harrington, & Howard, 2011). There is often overlap among these three services in terms of participants, providers, and services.

More than 2.8 million individuals were served through these Medicaid HCBS programs in 2007, having grown from 2.1 million in 2000. In 2007, almost 1.2 million individuals were served through HCBS waivers, 813,848 through the home health benefit, and 826,251 through the personal care services benefit, although it should be noted that individuals may be served in more than one program (Ng & Harrington, 2011). Overall, Medicaid LTC expenditures grew from $19 billion in 2000 to $42 billion in 2007 (Kitchener et al., 2005). By 2009, HCBS expenditures were more than $51 billion compared to $63 billion for institutional spending (Eiken, Sredl, Burwell, & Gold, 2010). In spite of the major increases in HCBS funding, some states are still reporting large waiting lists for HCBS waivers (366,000 in 2009), showing a large unmet need for services (Ng et al., 2011). The waiting lists, however, are highly variable from state to state and some states include individuals who have not been screened and may not qualify, while other states do not keep lists.

Federal Initiatives

Federal law has evolved to permit additional types of waivers and benefit programs to expand HCBS and to rebalance LTC spending from institutional services to HCBS. States have used the Section 1115 waiver program to implement managed care waivers. Arizona, Vermont, and Rhode Island use Section 1115 waivers to implement statewide Medicaid managed care programs that include HCBS (Crowley & O'Malley, 2008). In 2006, 16 states had approved Section 1115 waivers for Medicaid HCBS, and states continue to have access to Section 1115 waiver programs.

The Money Follows the Person (MFP) demonstrations were established under the Deficit Reduction Act (DRA) of 2005 for states to increase the use of community-based services with an enhanced federal medical assistance percentage (FMAP; i.e., matching rate) for 1 year for each person transitioned from an institution to the community (which was later extended). To be eligible, participants had to reside in an institution for a period from 6 months to 2 years. In 2007, there were 31 MFP grants awarded to states, with $1.4 billion in funds (Centers for Medicare and Medicaid Services [CMS], 2006). In 2009, 30 states had operational programs, and nearly 9,000 individuals had transitioned back to the community and another 4,000 transitions were in progress (Watts, 2011). In 2009, 29 states and the District of Columbia had MFP grants, and almost 6,000 individuals were returned to the community (CMS, Center for Medicaid, CHIP and Survey and Certification, & Mann, C., 2010a). In 2011, CMS approved 13 new state MFP grants (U.S. Department of Health & Human Services, 2011).

The DRA also established Section 1915(i) of the Social Security Act to allow states to offer HCBS as a state plan benefit as well as a 1915(c) waiver program. The benefit of the program was that states can offer HCBS to those who are not eligible for institutional services, which CMS calls breaking the "eligibility links." Individuals must meet specific needs-based criteria established by states that can be based on functional criteria such as activities of daily living or state risk factors. States can limit eligibility to specific geographic areas, to the categorically needy, and to specific services, with a renewal required every 5 years. States do not have to demonstrate that services cost the same or less than institutional services (as in the 1915(c) program). The legislation did not allow states to target the services to specific target populations, and the problematic part of the legislation was the limit on Medicaid eligibility to incomes not exceeding 150% of the federal poverty level (FPL; which is lower than the 300% of Supplemental Security Income allowed in the 1915(c) waiver program and for institutional care). Iowa was the first state to receive 1915(i) approval to offer statewide case management services and habilitation services to individuals needing psychiatric treatment (Sowers, 2008). Recently, Colorado, Nevada, Washington, and Wisconsin were approved for permanent waivers, and Idaho was approved for 5 years).

A Cash and Counseling option within the DRA, also known as 1915(j) state plan option, permits states to allow for self-direction of personal assistance services without needing to obtain a waiver. These include consumer protections consistent with the cash and counseling demonstration, prohibit individuals from participating in self-direction under the option if they live in a home or property owned or controlled by a service provider, and allow targeting of specific populations or regions of the states. Individuals may hire, fire, supervise, and manage service providers who may be family members. States could limit the number of enrollees who self-direct their care

(Carlson & Coffey, 2010). This option became effective in late 2007, and five states (Arkansas, Alabama, Oregon, New Jersey, and Florida) have approved 1915(j) options (Kaiser Family Foundation, 2006; Sowers, 2008), and more recently California, Louisiana, and New York were approved by CMS. The 1915(j) options are permanent.

ACA LEGISLATION

The ACA of 2010 contains three major provisions for the expansion of Medicaid HCBS. These are described and discussed separately in the following sections.

Community First Choice (CFC) Option

This CFC option provides a financial incentive to states to establish home- and community-based attendant supports and services (i.e., personal care services [PCS]) to individuals with disabilities (Section 2401), called 1915(k), starting October 1, 2011 (CMS, 2011a). It offers states an enhanced 6% federal medical assistance matching rate more than their current federal funds for personal attendant services, while states would be required to maintain their prior year expenditures for attendant services for the aged and disabled for 1 year (CMS, 2011a).

The law and the proposed CFC regulations state that eligibility for the program requires (a) being eligible for Medical assistance under the state plan and (b) having income that (1) is equal to or less than 150% of the (FPL) or (2) income over 150% of FPL and meets the state's eligibility criteria for institutional services (in a hospital, nursing facility, intermediate care facility for the mentally challenged, or an institution for mental diseases), or (3) qualifies for Medicaid under the state's special HCBS waiver criteria and is receiving at least one HCBS waiver service per month (CMS, 2011a). Optional Medicaid eligibility groups would include those categorized as working disabled who are eligible if their income is less than 250% of the FPL. The state must use the same income disregards they use under their Medicaid state plan.

Eligible individuals may choose to receive CFC attendant services and supports through a person-centered plan of care that meets the needs of the individual. Services must be provided in the most integrated setting appropriate to each care recipient. Providers must protect the health and welfare of enrollees, and individuals may use family members or others to provide the services if they meet the qualifications of the service plan.

Under the proposed CFC regulations, the state may choose to use one or more service delivery models: (1) "agency providers" that allow individual users or a user's representative to select, manage, and dismiss the provider (although providers are employed by the agency so the provider may continue to work for the agency) or (2) a "self-directed model" (CMS, 2011a). With respect to the agency model, states may allow services to be delivered through a traditional agency model or an agency with choice model, which allows a co-employment relationship between the individual and an agency. By contrast, the self-directed model is one that has a service plan and a service budget that individuals can use to meet their needs. Individuals can recruit, hire, fire, supervise, manage, and train workers; determine duties and schedules; evaluate performance; determine the amount paid for services; and review and approve provider invoices. The service budget must have a specific dollar amount set for the program and procedures to manage the funds. Other models may include the provision of vouchers, direct cash payments, or the use of a fiscal agent where providers are independent and services are consumer-controlled (CMS, 2011a).

The CFC scope of services allows for the acquisition, maintenance, and enhancement of skills necessary for the individual to accomplish tasks. Services may include the transition costs for moving from an institution to the home or community and other services to increase independence or substitute for human assistance. Excluded services are room and board costs, special education, assistive technology devices, medical supplies and equipment, and home modification (CMS, 2011a). Services and supports are intended to provide alternatives to institutional services and are not allowed in institutional settings where services are provided.

Each state must develop and implement a state plan amendment in collaboration with a development and implementation council with a majority of members with disabilities, elderly individuals, and their representatives. The program must be provided on a statewide basis without regard to restrictions by age, type/nature of disability, severity of disability, or the form of services required; the program would not be allowed to have waiting lists.

Other minimum CFC requirements include the establishment and maintenance of a comprehensive continuous quality assurance system; standards for training and services; systems for consumer feedback; monitoring the health of participants; mandatory data reporting, investigation, and resolution of complaints about abuse or neglect; information on the quality of services provided; federal reporting; and a program evaluation including information on the program quality and program choice. The program also must comply with the Fair Labor Standards Act of 1938, including the withholding and payment of income and payroll taxes, provision of unemployment and workers compensation insurance, maintenance of general liability insurance, and compliance with occupational health and safety.

The legislation requires that the Secretary of the Department of Health and Human Services conduct an evaluation of the CFC program, collect data on the program (including the number of individuals served, the characteristics of individuals in the program, and whether the individuals were previously served by other HCBS programs) and make an interim report to Congress in 2013 and a final report in 2015.

CRITIQUE

The CFC was designed to expand access to PCS, which are essential services for many individuals with disabilities who need assistance to maintain their daily functioning and to live at home and participate in the community. Although all states offered some types of HCBS 1915(c) waiver programs in 2010, 32 states had optional state plan personal care service programs, and 18 did not (see Table 1). All 18 states without state plan PCS offer some PCS through some of their 1915(c) waiver programs, but waiver participants must meet the institutional level of care criteria for eligibility, whereas the PCS state plan programs do not have to meet that level of need.

Many states recognize the importance of offering PCS, and three states have added the state plan PCS program in the past 5 years. Table 1 shows that states with the state plan PCS option generally have higher percentages of LTC expenditures devoted to HCBS than states that do not (the average is 48% vs. 40%, respectively). States currently without a PCS program that offer PCS through their waiver programs could shift these services to the new CFC program, and/or they could set up a new CFC program. One issue not clarified by CMS is whether states would want to and be allowed to shift their existing PCS programs to the new CFC program in order to obtain the higher federal matching assistance payment. In some ways, having a separate PCS program may simplify the administration of the 1915(c) waiver programs. On the other hand, adding a new PCS program in itself would add new state administrative structures.

There are disadvantages to using the CFC program from a state perspective. Probably the most important concern is that the state is required to offer PCS to all those who meet the eligibility requirements without geographic limits and the specific target group limits that the waivers can have. Under the waiver, states may also restrict participation and costs through waiting lists, but they will not be able to do so with the CFC option.

One area of concern is the eligibility criteria for the program. According to advocates, the intent of the legislation was to tie CFC eligibility to the state's institutional need criteria regardless of income eligibility (Oxford & Darling, 2011). In contrast, the proposed CFC regulations specifically allow states to provide CFC services to individuals earning less than 150% of the FPL without a level of care determination (CMS, 2011a). States may be reluctant to serve those earning less than 150% of the FPL without setting institution-level need requirements, although perhaps CMS will allow states to establish such criteria. Although it appears that individuals who are medically needy would be served if they meet the state's institutional need criteria, this was not clear in the proposed CFC regulations (CMS, 2011a).

TABLE 1 State Plan Personal Care Services Program Expenditures, Expenditures Per Capita, and Percentage of HCBS to Total Long Term Care in 2009

	Personal Care Expenditures	Personal Care per Capita	% HCBS to Total LTC
DC	$88,719,590	$147.95	51.4
NY	$2,721,249,447	$139.26	47.0
CA	$4,403,014,003	$119.12	58.7
AK	$82,371,964	$117.93	67.7
MA	$639,285,871	$96.96	48.0
MN	$409,853,665	$77.83	68.2
WA	$416,964,159	$62.57	66.2
NC	$525,600,917	$56.03	46.0
LA	$246,412,380	$54.85	38.8
MO	$317,985,287	$53.11	46.0
NM	$82,925,708	$41.26	83.4
NJ	$343,722,339	$39.47	30.5
ME	$50,823,033	$38.55	56.1
MT	$35,885,239	$36.81	49.5
WI	$179,328,014	$31.71	38.7
AR	$79,089,738	$27.37	33.7
MI	$261,855,273	$26.27	35.3
NV	$68,257,353	$25.82	46.8
ND	$13,991,476	$21.63	29.9
TX	$531,132,044	$21.43	45.9
WV	$38,238,959	$21.01	43.0
ID	$22,650,057	$14.65	47.9
NE	$15,539,899	$8.65	41.5
OR	$28,074,671	$7.34	73.3
MD	$35,070,139	$6.15	41.5
NH	$6,211,595	$4.69	44.0
OK	$11,747,333	$3.19	45.1
FL	$40,992,889	$2.21	35.6
SC	$9,817,657	$2.15	42.0
SD	$1,706,709	$2.10	41.1
AZ	$7,919,299	$1.20	N/A
KS	$2,766,929	$0.98	56.8
UT	$1,571,002	$0.56	45.8
GA	$622,959	$0.06	37.8
VA	$3,351	0	45.6
AL			31.0
CO			58.2
CT			46.2
DE			36.0
HI			54.8
IA			41.0
IL			29.6
IN			32.7
KY			33.1
MS			15.1
OH			35.7
PA			34.6
RI			46.5

(Continued)

TABLE 1 (Continued)

	Personal Care Expenditures	Personal Care per Capita	% HCBS to Total LTC
TN			35.2
VT			N/A
WY			57.9
US	$11,721,400,948	$38.18	44.8

Note. Source: Eiken et al., 2010.
AZ and VT do not have Medicaid 1915(c) waivers and the majority of the services are provided through a Section 1115 waiver.

The option adds a number of requirements for quality assurance, training standards, satisfaction and consumer feedback surveys, reporting requirements, and an evaluation that are not required for the waiver programs. These provisions rightfully are intended to create PCS programs that are more consumer-controlled. The requirement for states to establish consumer councils not required for the state PCS option or the HCBS waiver program may also be considered time-consuming and costly by states.

Some advocates have expressed concern that the proposed CFC regulations allow states to choose one or more service delivery models described as an agency model or a self-directed model with a service budget (CMS, 2011a). Advocates argue that the intent of the CFC option was to allow consumers maximum choice of using either an agency model or a self-directed model, so that consumer choice would be limited if CMS allows a state to elect only one model (Oxford & Darling, 2011). They have urged CMS to require states to offer both agency and self-directed models.

One major criticism of this option is that it remains optional rather than mandatory. Overall, the fear of new costs, administrative burdens, and limited staff resources may prevent states from taking advantage of the new CFC program. These concerns may override the 6% financial incentive offered by the new CFC option.

Amendments to the HCBS State Plan Benefit

Section 2402 of the ACA amended the Section 1915(i) optional HCBS state plan benefit established under the DRA. First, it allows the state to serve individuals with incomes up to 300% of the Supplemental Security Income payment rate (rather than 150% of the FPL). The 300% eligibility, however, is limited only to those individuals eligible for an existing waiver (i.e., 1915(c), (d), or (e) or 1115). Furthermore, states can use the institutional eligibility and post-eligibility rules that specify the share of costs individuals must pay for services in the community. States must also project the number of individuals expected to receive the services each year and submit data on the number served. States can expand Medicaid eligibility for categorically eligible persons (ie, who qualify because they are eligible for Supplemental Security Income programs) but they can exclude individuals who are medically needy (ie, those who have medical expenses that reduce their incomes to the state Medicaid eligibility levels) (Carlson & Coffey, 2010).

Second, the legislation removes the "statewide" exemption (the requirement that all individuals throughout a state who are eligible for a benefit must receive the benefit) and removes the enrollment caps of 1915(i) waivers. In other words, it eliminated the option to limit the number of eligible individuals in the program except by establishing needs-based eligibility criteria, or the length of time that individuals may be grandfathered if the eligibility criteria are modified. Third, it permits states to extend full Medicaid benefits to individuals receiving HCBS under a state plan and expands the type, amount, duration, or scope of services that can be offered. It also allows states to extend full Medicaid benefits to individuals who meet the requirements for the 1915(i) program (Stone et al., 2010).

Fourth, states can target particular groups of people and establish needs-based eligibility criteria for the groups that were specified (CMS, Center for Medicaid, CHIP and Survey and Certification, Mann, C., 2010b). States are allowed to revise the needs-based criteria by giving a 60-day public notice without CMS approval, although they must continue to serve those individuals who do not meet the new revised needs criteria as long as the state HCBS option is authorized. States, however, must demonstrate that the needs-based criteria for the 1915(i) program are less stringent than the state's institutional level of care criteria (CMS et al., 2010b).

Finally, states are allowed to have "targeted benefits" for specific population groups. For example, states can have one benefit for those with physical and/or developmental disabilities and other benefits for those with chronic mental illness, children, or HIV/AIDS, as long as the services meet the needs for each target population group (CMS et al., 2010b). Basic services include case management, homemaker/home health aide, personal care, adult day health, habilitation, and respite care. Additional services may be provided for those with chronic mental illness including day treatment, partial hospitalization, psychosocial rehabilitation, and clinic services. States may also offer other services as requested (but not room and board).

The program can continue to offer self-directed services to allow participants to plan and purchase services under their direction or through an authorized representative, based on an individualized plan of care that is based on an independent assessment and a person-centered process of care. These new provisions were effective October 1, 2010 (42 CFR 430.12(e)(i)), and states had to submit a state plan amendment by December 31, 2010 (CMS et al., 2010b).

CRITIQUE

These new amendments are a step forward in correcting some of the limitations of the DRA, especially the financial eligibility limitation of 150% of the FPL. Since most waivers had a 300% of Supplemental Security Income eligibility level set by the state, the lower threshold was a limitation for converting to the state plan.

The HCBS state plan option is attractive because the option can be renewed after 5 years and it eliminates meeting the cost neutrality provisions required under the HCBS 1915(c) waivers. By giving states flexibility in the number and types of services offered and the targeted population groups, the ACA allows states to consolidate their 1915(c) waivers. This HCBS state plan option is consistent with new 2011 proposed CMS regulatory changes to the 1915(c) waivers program (CMS, 2011b). Under this new proposed regulation, the 1915(c) waiver program could use one combined waiver to serve persons who are (1) aged or disabled or both, (2) mentally challenged or developmentally disabled or both, and (3) mentally ill (CMS, 2011b), although the waivers would continue to have all their existing requirements for cost neutrality.

Some states have many 1915(c) waivers (Colorado, Texas, and Wisconsin = 12; Florida = 14; New York and Pennsylvania = 13; Eiken et al., 2010), and each one generally has its own administrative structure, screening tools and needs criteria, and benefits. The administrative costs and the variations across waivers could probably be reduced significantly by combining the programs under one state plan option. By consolidating the waivers into a new HCBS state plan program and avoiding the federal paperwork and the cost neutrality requirements of waivers, states may be able to improve access to services while reducing costs.

At the same time, each of the waivers has developed its own constituent groups. If the program is changed from a waiver to a state plan benefit, constituent groups may become concerned that services might be reduced to their particular group and try to block changes through political action. Moreover, administrative units within states may not wish to change their current program structure. Internal state politics can be a major barrier to structural change.

State Balancing Incentive Program

This program (Section 10202) is titled "Incentives for States to Offer Home and Community-Based Services as a Long-Term Care Alternative to Nursing Homes" and provides enhanced federal matching payments to eligible states to increase the proportion of spending on all LTC services that are non–institutionally-based (i.e., HCBS) over 4 years starting in October 2011. Non–institutionally-based LTC services are defined as home health care services, personal care services, PACE program services, and self-directed personal assistance services.

The program applies to states that spend less than 50% of their LTC expenditures on HCBS. States that spent less than 25% of their total LTC expenditures in FY 2009 on HCBS, if they apply for this program, would be required to increase HCBS spending to 25% by 2015. These states would receive an increase in federal Medicaid match for HCBS of five percentage points. In states with between 25% and 50% HCBS spending, the state target requirement would be to spend 50% by 2015, and these states would receive a two–percentage point increase in federal match. States are required not to make eligibility for HCBS more restrictive than the eligibility standards, methods, and procedures in force on December 31, 2010.

The state is required to submit an application for the incentive program with a proposed budget to expand and diversify the HCBS program. If the state proposes to expand the HCBS under the 1915(i) program, the state should increase the income eligibility from 150% of the FPL to 300% of the Supplemental Security Income benefit to meet the requirement for the incentive program. The state would be required to agree to use the additional matching federal funds only on providing new or expanded HCBS services.

Within 6 months of approval, the state would be required to enact three structural program changes. First, the state would establish a "no wrong door–single entry point system," which would coordinate all LTC services and supports through an agency, organization, network, or portal for providing information on availability of services, referral services, assistance with procedures, and determinations of both financial and functional eligibility for services. Second, the state would provide "conflict-free case management services," which usually means having a single case manager directing care and working with other providers or specialists to assure that multiple case managers are not billing or directing care for the individual. It could also mean that entities conducting the assessment of need and developing the service plan are not related, are not financially responsible, or would not benefit from the assessment and management of services, as defined in the CFC regulations (CMS, 2011a). The service plan, arrangement of services and supports in directing services, and monitoring of services are delivered to meet the beneficiaries' needs and achieve intended outcomes.

Third, standardized assessment instruments must be used for determining eligibility for HCBS and supports to meet the needs for training, support services, medical care, transportation, and other services. Finally, the state would agree to collect data from providers on individual use of HCBS and supports, a core set of quality measures on population specific outcomes, and outcome data on beneficiary and family caregiver experience with providers, satisfaction with services, and desired outcomes such as employment, community participation, health, and prevention of loss in function. The total of all incentive payments made to states is limited to $3 billion.

CRITIQUE

This program is targeted to rebalancing HCBS against institutional care in the states with the lowest proportionate HCBS spending. Table 2 shows that only one state (Mississippi) had less than 25% of total LTC expenditures on HCBS and 35 states had between 25% and 50% according to data compiled by Thomson Reuters. (Arizona and Vermont provide LTC expenditures in 1115 waivers so their data are not complete.) This option should be attractive to states interested in improving their HCBS balance without having to add a new statewide program that the CFC would require.

If the rebalancing provisions applied specifically to the Medicaid aged and disabled population, which is more at risk of nursing home placement, 24 states would be able to qualify for the higher 5% FMAP because they have less than 25% of LTC expenditures for HCBS, and all but six states would be eligible for the program because they have 25% to 50% of total LTC expenditures for HCBS (See Table 2, column 5). Congress may have intended the funds to be used for the rebalancing of the aged and disabled population in particular (which is suggested by the section title that mentions nursing homes specifically) rather than the entire LTC population. This would obviously increase the costs of the program since more states would qualify for funds.

A key question is whether the incentive levels are sufficient to encourage many states to commit to the increased spending on HCBS required over a 5-year period. States have many reasons to accept the incentive offer. Many have long waiting lists of eligible individuals who want to use HCBS services. Moreover, several states have Olmstead litigation pending (currently there are more than 40 active or unsettled Olmstead cases in 24 states; Center for Personal Assistance Services, 2011).

On the other hand, the structural changes required by the incentive program are substantial. Setting up a single entry point system, which has important benefits for individual consumers, requires redesign of existing state programs to consolidate and make the entry point administrative units accessible to consumers. Although most states see the value of independent case management (separate from providers) to reduce conflicts of interest and to control admission assessments, reassessments, and service authorizations, this requirement could involve hiring new state staff or contracting out case management services. The conflict-free case management provision that prohibits those who make client assessments and service plans from benefiting financially could affect managed care organizations that may have a conflict.

State officials may see the advantage of standardized assessment instruments for determining eligibility for services; however, making changes in instruments can affect many different programs and constituency groups. California, for example, has made efforts to use standardized instruments

TABLE 2 Proportion of Medicaid HCBS Expenditures of Total Medicaid LTC Expenditures in 2009 and FMAP under the HCBS Incentive Benefit of the ACA

	HCBS 2009[1]	LTC 2009[1]	% Total HCBS/LTC[1]	% Aged Disabled HCBS/LTC[1]	Regular FMAP[2]	Enhanced FMAP
AK	$252,561,562	$372,871,901	67.7	55.7	0.5053	0.5053
AL	$438,806,576	$1,414,860,887	31.0	14.9	0.6798	0.6998
AR	$365,276,497	$1,082,471,177	33.7	29.0	0.7281	0.7481
AZ	$9,033,182	$42,152,650	N/A	N/A	0.6577	
CA	$6,517,886,786	$11,097,802,261	58.7	55.1	0.5000	0.5000
CO	$797,996,360	$1,370,380,509	58.2	43.6	0.5000	0.5000
CT	$1,516,168,534	$3,280,286,895	46.2	24.3	0.5000	0.5200
DC	$286,662,072	$557,724,202	51.4	45.6	0.7000	0.7000
DE	$120,014,480	$333,763,098	36.0	12.5	0.5000	0.5200
FL	$1,507,068,472	$4,237,877,425	35.6	20.5	0.5540	0.5740
GA	$748,012,573	$1,977,131,027	37.8	26.0	0.6449	0.6649
HI	$139,073,151	$253,736,770	54.8	19.2	0.5511	0.5511
IA	$532,145,157	$1,298,260,032	41.0	29.6	0.6262	0.6462
ID	$194,964,284	$407,447,615	47.9	43.3	0.6977	0.7177
IL	$916,517,066	$3,093,396,517	29.6	19.8	0.5032	0.5232
IN	$740,060,814	$2,262,531,084	32.7	16.2	0.6426	0.6626
KS	$579,383,292	$1,020,745,285	56.8	39.4	0.6008	0.6008
KY	$459,366,913	$1,387,667,418	33.1	19.3	0.7013	0.7213
LA	$767,292,107	$1,979,606,248	38.8	32.5	0.7131	0.7331
MA	$1,739,056,166	$3,620,676,478	48.0	35.9	0.5000	0.5200
MD	$784,496,744	$1,890,176,998	41.5	14.9	0.5000	0.5200
ME	$405,782,955	$722,900,885	56.1	24.5	0.6441	0.6441
MI	$837,890,881	$2,376,290,776	35.3	21.5	0.6027	0.6227
MN	$2,164,351,802	$3,175,806,702	68.2	57.5	0.5000	0.5000
MO	$870,174,316	$1,893,231,018	46.0	33.7	0.6319	0.6519
MS	$178,917,475	$1,183,463,101	15.1	15.8	0.7584	0.8084
MT	$166,786,079	$337,223,441	49.5	33.9	0.6804	0.7004
NC	$1,530,426,971	$3,329,404,170	46.0	42.8	0.6460	0.6660
ND	$107,501,966	$359,330,237	29.9	10.2	0.6315	0.6515
NE	$273,186,838	$658,113,063	41.5	24.9	0.5954	0.6154
NH	$249,996,686	$567,868,863	44.0	17.7	0.5000	0.5200
NJ	$1,146,377,769	$3,754,425,268	30.5	21.2	0.5000	0.5200
NM	$419,908,376	$503,643,718	83.4	68.8	0.7088	0.7088
NV	$157,082,327	$335,824,047	46.8	34.1	0.5000	0.5200
NY	$9,506,953,405	$20,237,825,602	47.0	38.1	0.5000	0.5200
OH	$1,803,755,463	$5,051,981,260	35.7	24.1	0.6214	0.6414
OK	$539,127,664	$1,194,837,905	45.1	32.4	0.6590	0.6790
OR	$958,979,907	$1,307,892,511	73.3	56.2	0.6245	0.6245
PA	$2,234,687,629	$6,458,078,101	34.6	17.9	0.5452	0.5652
RI	$265,920,855	$571,404,796	46.5	4.4	0.5259	0.5459
SC	$491,575,117	$1,171,352,627	42.0	27.9	0.7007	0.7207
SD	$115,695,916	$281,302,839	41.1	14.0	0.6255	0.6455
TN	$674,182,772	$1,916,773,226	35.2	8.9	0.6428	0.6628
TX	$2,584,970,257	$5,635,627,491	45.9	44.5	0.5944	0.6144
UT	$177,905,204	$388,360,081	45.8	19.6	0.7071	0.7271
VA	$883,322,914	$1,935,928,364	45.6	35.1	0.5000	0.5200
VT	$56,856,875	$175,071,974	N/A	N/A	0.5945	

(*Continued*)

TABLE 2 (Continued)

	HCBS 2009[1]	LTC 2009[1]	% Total HCBS/LTC[1]	% Aged Disabled HCBS/LTC[1]	Regular FMAP[2]	Enhanced FMAP
WA	$1,447,943,331	$2,186,657,594	66.2	62.0	0.5094	0.5094
WI	$873,203,370	$2,255,268,605	38.7	26.0	0.5938	0.6138
WV	$394,606,696	$917,893,880	43.0	25.5	0.7373	0.7573
WY	$124,489,528	$214,845,338	57.9	23.4	0.5000	0.5000
US	$51,054,404,132	$114,080,193,960	44.8	33.8		

Note. Sources: Eiken et al., 2010; Kaiser Family Foundation, 2010.
AZ and VT do not have Medicaid 1915(c) waivers, and the majority of the services are provided through a Section 1115 waiver.

for almost 20 years without being able to obtain the agreement of program officials, advocacy groups, and providers. Moreover, the program's reporting requirements may also be viewed as a barrier by some states.

The outcome goals for this program may be difficult to achieve. It is a much further stretch for a state to go from 26% to reach the 50% goal than it is for other states that are closer to the goal to begin with. Another approach would have been to set a percentage improvement goal, such as a 25% improvement in the state's HCBS proportion spent on LTC expenditures, and this would have allowed more states to participate in this option.

Other ACA Changes

The law extended the Medicaid MFP program through 2016 with $2.25 billion in funding. The law allows individuals who have been in the facility for a period "not less than 90 consecutive days" to be transitioned from institutions, rather than the previous 6-month requirement (Section 2403(2)(b)). States must continue to provide community services after the demonstration period for as long as the individual remains on Medicaid and in need of community services. In 2011, CMS approved 13 new states to join the 29 states and the District of Columbia that already have MFP grants (U.S. Department of Health & Human Services, 2011). Existing MFP grants can be extended, and CMS will allow for new applications from states not currently participating. Finally, the ACA allocated $10 million per year for 5 years to continue funding Aging and Disability Resource Centers.

The ACA also mandates that the current spousal impoverishment protections be applied to beneficiaries who qualify for Medicaid HCBS, in addition to those who qualify for Medicaid nursing home benefits, but is not effective until 2014 and then is limited to a 5-year period. This includes individuals who are eligible for HCBS under 1915 sections (c), (d), and (i) and waivers under Section 1115, the medically needy, and those receiving services under Section 1915(k), the CFC option (ACA, Section 2404). States are already able to use the spousal impoverishment provisions under the current 1915(c) waiver program regulations as an option, but it is not mandatory.

This spousal impoverishment provision will improve access to HCBS for those with income and assets previously precluded from participation. Delaying the effective date probably was done for financial reasons, but it places an unfair limitation on those who elect HCBS over institutional services. Moreover, the 5-year limit allows time to assess the financial impact of the legislation while at the same time creating uncertainty for states as well as individual users.

IMPLICATIONS

The ACA introduces three programs that should be attractive to states that want to expand HCBS services, and two have important financial incentives. The three programs also have barriers that may limit the willingness of states to adopt the programs at this time, discussed above. If states have to adopt structural changes in the state administration of HCBS programs and to accept more reporting requirements, they may be unwilling to do so.

State budgetary problems are also critical to whether states are willing to expand HCBS services. After a severe recession, 48 states reported large shortfalls in 2009 and 2010 because of a sharp decline in tax receipts and a growing demand for state-funded services (McNichol, Oliff, & Johnson, 2010). In 2010, 46 states reported $130 billion (20%) in shortfalls, and these problems are not expected to diminish even by 2012, when 40 states are projecting shortfalls (McNichol et al., 2010). These budget crises place severe pressure on states to cut services. The AARP (2011) survey of states found that 31 states reported cutting non-Medicaid aging and disability services in 2010, and 28 states were expecting to cut the programs in 2011. Most states cut Medicaid provider rates and some cut services, particularly personal care services, at a time when the demand for services was increased (AARP Public Policy Institute, 2011). The survey found that 35 states reported increases in HCBS waiver programs from 2009 to 2011, and 22 states expected the number of nursing home residents to decline while 12 states expected the number to stay the same (AARP Public Policy Institute, 2011). Moreover, the nursing home industry has more political power in lobbying for scarce state resources than HCBS providers. Clearly, the budget constraints place pressures on states to control or reduce LTC expenditures and place HCBS in direct competition with institutional services.

One issue is, What should be the targets that states can reach in rebalancing? Eiken et al. (2010) reported that New Mexico spent 83% of total LTC dollars on HCBS in 2009 (Table 2). Oregon spent 73% of its total Medicaid LTC expenditures on HCBS but 99% of its LTC funds for the developmentally disabled on HCBS and 56% of LTC funds for the aged and disabled on

HCBS. Michigan, Alaska, and New Hampshire spent 98% of LTC on HCBS for individuals with developmental disabilities. All states spent an average 34% of LTC funds on HCBS for the aged and disabled but 66% of HCBS funds for the developmentally disabled (data not shown; Eiken et al., 2010). Clearly, some states have made remarkable progress in shifting LTC dollars to HCBS. Progress has been especially strong for individuals with developmental disabilities in part by closing large state facilities and shifting individuals to HCBS. However, the pressing issue is that many states need to work on targeting a higher proportion of the aged and disabled populations for HCBS, especially as the population ages.

The major provisions to expand HCBS are voluntary, with federal incentives to encourage change. Congress has been unwilling to make HCBS mandatory and to set standards for access to HCBS, while current law has mandatory requirements for institutional services. Without minimum standards for HCBS services, the wide variations across states will continue to occur. These variations range from three HCBS participants per 1,000 population in Georgia to 15 in Washington, DC, with an average of nine HCBS participants per 1,000 population in 2007 (Ng & Harrington, 2011). HCBS expenditures vary from $486 per capita in New York to $59 in Nevada in 2009 (Eiken et al., 2010). Moreover, there is no requirement to cover all target groups (such as children, people with HIV/AIDS, and people with traumatic brain or spinal cord injuries) so unmet needs occur for special populations. In other states, the majority of expenditures are targeted to individuals with developmental disabilities with limited expenditures for other groups. As long as states have the option to deny Medicaid HCBS to people who meet the criteria for institutional services, access and financial inequities will continue.

REFERENCES

AARP Public Policy Institute. (2011). *Weathering the storm: The impact of the great recession on long-term services and supports*. In Brief 188. Washington, DC: AARP. January.

Carlson, E., & Coffey, G. (2010). *10-plus years after the Olmstead ruling*. Washington, DC: National Senior Citizens Law Center. September.

Center for Personal Assistance Services. (2011). *State Olmstead litigation*. San Francisco, CA: University of California. Retrieved from http://www.pascenter.org/state_based_stats/pick_a_state.php?url=http%3A%2F%2Fwww.pascenter.org%2Fstate_based_stats%2Folmstead_home.php&title=Olmstead+Decision+and+Lawsuits+by+State

Centers for Medicare and Medicaid Services, Center for Medicaid, CHIP and Survey and Certification, Mann, C. (2010a). *Extension of the Money Follows the Person rebalancing demonstration program, memo to state Medicaid directors, SMDL # 10–012*, Baltimore, MD: CMS. June 22.

Centers for Medicare and Medicaid Services, Center for Medicaid, CHIP and Survey and Certification, Mann., C. (2010b). *Improving access to home and community based services, memo to state Medicaid directors, SMDL # 10–013*, Baltimore, MD: CMS, August 6.

Centers for Medicare and Medicaid Services (CMS). (2011a). Medicaid program: Community First Choice option. 42 CFR Part 441. Proposed rule. *Federal Register, 76*(38), 10736–10753, February 25.

Centers for Medicare and Medicaid Services (CMS). (2011b). Medicaid program: Home and community-based services (HCBS) waivers. 42 CFR Part 441 Proposed Rule. *Federal Register, 76*(73), 21311–21317, April 15.

Centers for Medicare and Medicaid Services (CMS). (2006). *Money Follows the Person rebalancing demonstration. funding opportunity.* No. HHS-2007-CMS-RCMFTP-0003, DHHS. Retrieved from www.cms.hhs.gov/NewFreedomInitiative/downloads/MFP_2007_Announcement.pdf

Crowley, J., & O'Malley, M. (2008). *Vermont's choices for care Medicaid long-term services waiver: Progress and challenges as the program concluded its third year.* Washington, DC: The Kaiser Commission on Medicaid and the Uninsured, November.

Eiken, S., Sredl, K., Burwell, B., & Gold, L. (2010). *Medicaid LTC expenditures in FY 2009.* Cambridge, MA: Thomson Reuters.

Hartman, M., Martin, A., McDonnell, P., Catlin, A., & National Health Expenditure Accounts Team. (2009). National health spending in 2007: Slower drug spending contributes to lowest rate of overall growth since 1998. *Health Affairs, 28*(1), 46–261.

Kaiser Family Foundation. (2006). *Medicaid long-term services reforms in the Deficit Reduction Act.* Washington, DC: Kaiser. Retrieved from http://www.kff.org/medicaid/7486.cfm

Kaiser Family Foundation. (2010). *Federal Medical Assistance Percentage (FMAP) for Medicaid with American Recovery and Reinvestment Act (ARRA) adjustments. ARRA rates quarter 4, 2010.* Washington, DC: Kaiser. Retrieved from http://www.statehealthfacts.org/comparemaptable.jsp?ind=695&cat=4&sort=a&gsa=2

Kitchener, M., Ng, T., & Harrington, C. (2007). Medicaid state plan personal care services: Trends in programs and policies. *Journal of Health and Social Policy, 19*(3), 9–26.

Kitchener, M., Ng, T., Miller, N., & Harrington, C. (2005). Medicaid home and community-based services: National program trends. *Health Affairs, 24*(1), 206–212.

McNichol, E., Oliff, P., & Johnson, N. (2010). *States continue to feel recession's impact.* Washington, DC: Center of Budget and Policy Priorities. December.

Ng, T., & Harrington, C. (2011). *State options that expand access to Medicaid home- and community-based services.* Menlo Park, CA: Kaiser Commission on Medicaid and the Uninsured.

Ng, T., Harrington, C., & Howard, J. (2011). *Medicaid home- and community-based service programs: Data update.* Menlo Park, CA: Kaiser Commission on Medicaid and the Uninsured.

Oxford, M., & Darling, B. (2011). *ADAPT's comments on the Centers for Medicare and Medicaid Services' proposed rules for "Medicaid programs: Community First Choice option."* 42 CFR Part 441, CMS-2337-P, RIN 0938-AQ35. Unpublished letter. Topeka, KS: ADAPT, April 7.

Sowers, M. (2008). *Home- and community-based services: 1915(c), 1915(i), and 1915(j).* Presented at the 2008 National Home and Community Based Conference, Boston, MA.

Stone, J., Baumrucker, E., Binder, C., Herz, E., Heisler, E., & Rothenburger, A. (2010). *Medicaid and the state children's health insurance program (CHIP) provision in PPACA: summary and timeline.* Report 7–5700. Washington, DC: Congressional Research Service.

U.S. Department of Health & Human Services. (2011). *Affordable Care Act supports states in strengthening home and community-based services* [news release]. Washington, DC: Retrieved from www.hhs.gov/news/press/2011pres/02/20110222b.html

Watts, M. O. (2011). *Money Follows the Person: A 2010 snapshot.* Washington, DC: Kaiser Commission on Medicaid and the Uninsured. Retrieved from http://www.kff.org/medicaid/8141.cfm

The Impact of Health Care Reform on the Workforce Caring for Older Adults

ROBYN I. STONE, DrPH

Executive Director, LeadingAge Center for Applied Research, Washington, District of Columbia, USA

NATASHA BRYANT, MA

Senior Research Associate, LeadingAge Center for Applied Research, Washington, District of Columbia, USA

This article summarizes the Patient Protection and Affordable Care Act (ACA) provisions that have a direct or indirect impact on the workforce caring for the elder population, explores the challenges to developing the workforce, and critiques the adequacy of the ACA provisions in meeting those challenges. The ACA is the first comprehensive federal legislation to acknowledge gaps in the workforce caring for the elder population. However, its provisions are inadequate given insufficient supply in the number and types of workers necessary both to meet the caregiving demand of the growing elder population and to implement the delivery system reforms instituted by the ACA. One of the challenges is that the workforce is not prepared for the new service delivery models specified in the legislation. They are not trained, supported, or held accountable for effective care coordination and service integration, and they lack the requisite skills, knowledge, and competencies. Moreover, it is likely to remain difficult to recruit and retain competent direct care workers, who represent the largest component of the long-term care workforce, because of the negative industry image, noncompetitive wages and benefits, a challenging work environment, and inadequate education and training. Several of the ACA provisions for developing the workforce have not received appropriations. Most are also demonstration projects of limited scope and duration.

INTRODUCTION

The Patient Protection and Affordable Care Act (ACA) includes a number of provisions designed to radically transform the way in which services and supports for older people are paid for and delivered. Successful implementation of these reforms will require a substantially different health and long-term care workforce than exists today. This elder care workforce includes the full range of health professionals who provide elder care: physicians, nurses, social workers, pharmacists, therapists, and other allied health professionals. It also includes direct care workers—nursing assistants, home health care aides, home care/personal care aides—who, next to family members, provide the lion's share of long-term care to older adults who are disabled and chronically ill.

This article begins with a brief summary of the key ACA provisions that have direct or indirect impacts on the elder care workforce. This is followed by a discussion of the workforce challenges and a critical review of the adequacy of these provisions in addressing the supply and demand issues associated with the aging of the population and the delivery system changes instituted by the ACA. The article concludes by observing that the ACA is groundbreaking legislation in its explicit attention to the need for a quality, competent workforce to meet the demands of an aging society. At the same time, without adequate funding for the workforce provisions included in health care reform and a specific focus within the payment/delivery system reforms on investments in ongoing education and better compensation, the ACA is unlikely to have a significant impact on the development and sustainability of this workforce.

ACA PROVISIONS TARGETED TO THE WORKFORCE

Provisions Directly Focused on Developing and Expanding the Workforce

A number of ACA provisions directly affect the development of the workforce caring for the elder population. These include the establishment of several oversight commissions and a national infrastructure for health care workforce development, payment incentives, expanded education and training initiatives, and other incentives to increase the supply.

WORKFORCE DEVELOPMENT INFRASTRUCTURE

The ACA authorized the creation of a 15-member national commission, the National Health Care Workforce Commission, to review projected workforce needs, recommend ways to align federal healthcare workforce resources to meet the demand, communicate and coordinate with various departments in the federal executive branch, and assess reports generated by the National Center for Health Care Workforce Analysis. The National Center for Health Care Workforce Analysis was established by the ACA to describe and analyze the health care workforce on a periodic basis. The Center has an authorization of $7.5 million dollars annually for FY 2010 through 2014. State and regional centers were also authorized at funding levels of $4.5 million annually for FY 2010 through 2014. The legislation established a grants program to enable state- and local-level partnerships to develop strategies for health care workforce development and to support innovative approaches to increase the number of skilled health care workers. Another provision created a Personal Care Attendants Advisory Panel tasked with advising the Secretary of the Department of Health and Human Services on how to address challenges to creating a quality, stable personal care workforce, including adequacy of the supply of these caregivers, their wages and benefits, and consumer access to their services.

PAYMENT INCENTIVES

One ACA provision that augments payments to primary care clinicians serving Medicare beneficiaries has the potential to expand the workforce caring for the elder population. Beginning in 2011, for a period of 5 years, Medicare will pay a 10% bonus for office visits, nursing facility visits, and home visits by primary care physicians, nurse practitioners, clinical nurse specialists, or physician assistants practicing family medicine, internal medicine, geriatrics, or pediatrics (Abrams, Nuzum, Mika, & Lawlor, 2011). The ACA invests an estimated $3.5 billion in the primary care provider bonus program from 2011 to 2016.

HEALTH CARE PROFESSIONALS TRAINING AND SUPPORT

The ACA includes a number of reforms intended to expand the supply of geriatrically trained health professionals. It authorized $10.8 million to geriatric education centers to support training in geriatrics, chronic-care management, and long-term care for faculty in health professions schools, including the development of curricula and best practices in geriatrics. The health care reform legislation authorized the expansion of the Geriatric Career Incentive Award program to encourage advance practice nurses, clinical social workers, pharmacists, and psychologists to pursue education and training leading to a career in care for elders and created a parallel Geriatrics Career Incentive Award program for master's-level candidates ($10 million over 3 years). The ACA also established targeted traineeships for advanced practice nurses who are pursuing careers in long-term care, geropsychiatric nursing, or other nursing areas that specialize in care of the elder population. Another provision increased the loan amounts in the nursing student loan program and specifically identified long-term care as one of the priority areas. Additionally, the ACA removed caps on awards for nurses pursuing advanced degrees in geriatrics. This legislation established a demonstration program to increase graduate nurse education training under Medicare that will provide advance practice nurses with the skills necessary to deliver primary and preventive care, transitional care, chronic-care management, and other nursing services appropriate for the Medicare-eligible population. An annual appropriation from the Medicare Hospital Insurance Trust Fund of $50 million was authorized for FY 2010 through 2015. Finally, the ACA required federally funded geriatric education centers to provide at least two courses each year, at no charge or nominal cost and in collaboration with appropriate community partners, to family caregivers who support frail older adults and individuals with disabilities.

DIRECT CARE WORKER TRAINING

The ACA included specific provisions designed to strengthen the competency of the direct care workforce. First, the act authorized $10 million over 3 years for new training opportunities for direct care workers. Grants are available to eligible entities for training of direct care workers employed in long-term care settings, such as nursing homes, assisted living communities, and home care settings. Once training is completed, the trainee must work in the field of geriatrics, disability services, long-term care, or chronic care management for a minimum of 2 years. In addition, the ACA authorized $67.5 million in grants and incentives to enhance training, recruitment, and retention of direct care staff (including career ladders and wage/benefit increases) and improve management practices affecting retention in either long-term care organizations or community-based programs or settings. Among these is a demonstration program that awards grants to up to six states for 3 years to develop 10 core competencies for personal or home care aides. The grantees must demonstrate approaches to implementing training that advances the core competencies and to developing training protocols, including a certification test for personal or home care aides who have completed the core competency training. An evaluation of the program will examine the impact of the core training on mastery of the personal aides' job skills, their job satisfaction, and beneficiary and family satisfaction with services and supports. Finally, the ACA required dementia and abuse prevention modules to be included in the national minimum requirement of 75 hours of pre-employment training for individuals interested in becoming certified nurse aides.

QUALITY MONITORING

The ACA includes three provisions designed to help promote and monitor the quality of the long-term care workforce. The first, part of a set of nursing home transparency provisions, requires the federal government to implement a system to collect and report information about how well nursing homes are staffed, including accurate information about the hours of service residents receive, staff turnover rates, and how much facilities spend on wages and benefits. The second provision extends to all states an existing pilot program that enables states to conduct national background checks, including fingerprint checks, on individuals who apply for direct patient access jobs in nursing homes and other long-term care facilities and with home care agencies that receive funding from Medicare or Medicaid. This provision is designed to eliminate the ability of persons with criminal histories to move from state to state to work with vulnerable older adults. The federal government is required to provide federal matching funds to states that choose to participate, and the checks should be implemented in such a way that does not result in application fees for long-term care workers. Currently, the Centers for Medicaid and Medicare Services has made $3 million available to 14 states that have chosen to participate in the program. The ACA also authorized the Secretary of the U.S. Department of Health and Human Services, in consultation with appropriate agencies and private sector organizations, to conduct a study on establishing a national nurse registry.

Other Provisions Influencing the Workforce

The ACA indirectly influences the workforce through the expansion of health insurance coverage and creation of delivery system reforms, which are described in more detail in other articles in this issue. The ACA expands health insurance coverage to all Americans through extending the Medicaid program to all adults who earn less than 133% of the federal poverty level (FPL) and helping individuals with incomes between 133% and 400% of the FPL to purchase private insurance through an insurance exchange (PHI, 2011). The legislation encourages and supports better service coordination and integration by establishing two new offices in the Centers for Medicare and Medicaid Services and the creation of several demonstration programs. It also created accountable care organizations (ACOs), which will be charged with managing the health care needs of a minimum of

5,000 Medicare beneficiaries for at least 3 years (McClellan, McKethan, Lewis, Roski, & Fisher, 2010). Under ACOs, providers of varying types will be held jointly accountable for the quality of the health care provided while keeping costs down. Several other ACA provisions were designed to help transform the delivery of long term services and supports to the disabled elder population and younger people with disabilities primarily through expanding home- and community-based services options (Justice, 2010).

WORKFORCE IMPLICATIONS

The ACA is the first comprehensive federal legislation to acknowledge gaps in the workforce caring for the elder population. The specific provisions designed to help increase the number and range of geriatrically trained health care professionals and direct care workers, in particular, is unprecedented. At the same time, concerns remain about the adequacy of these provisions in light of the aging of the population over the next 20 years and the delivery system reforms included in the ACA.

Challenges to Developing the Professional Health Care Workforce and Limits of the ACA

Workforce ill-prepared in competencies, knowledge, and skills for new service delivery models

The new models of service delivery outlined in the ACA require that staff in each setting and across settings understand how to coordinate and integrate care at the organizational level and at the individual patient/consumer level. Today's health care workforce is woefully ill-prepared and does not have the financial and organizational support—including the appropriate education and training—to implement the new service delivery models specified in the ACA. They lack the requisite knowledge, skills, and competencies, including the ability to organize and work in interdisciplinary teams, to document and share clinical information in a timely fashion within their own organizations, let alone across settings; to adequately address the complex issues that arise when individuals transfer from one setting to another; and to place the elder consumer (and family member where applicable) in the center of care decisions (Counsell et al., 2007). Even if the financial incentives across payers and providers were perfectly aligned, there is no guarantee that the clinicians, managerial staff, and direct care workers know how to use these integrated funds in the most appropriate and efficient manner to achieve better quality of care and quality of life for the care recipients, and at lower cost. Perhaps most important, better care coordination and integration cannot be achieved by staff with little to no experience in how effectively to incorporate the consumer and family members into the many decision-making processes that occur over time.

Some have suggested that the hospital with extended hospital medical staff (a concentrated group of physicians who work with and admit to their local hospital) is a prime candidate for becoming an ACO that would improve care coordination and achieve better care quality at a lower cost (Fisher, Staiger, Bynum, & Gottlieb, 2007). However, existing hospitals and local admitting physicians would not necessarily begin to practice care in a more coordinated fashion just by realigning the financial incentives and creating an ACO structure. Some have argued that providing higher-quality, more cost-effective care to older people with chronic conditions "will require aggressive initiatives to educate primary care physicians to apply principles of geriatrics—for example, optimizing functional autonomy and quality of life—within emerging models of chronic care" (Boult et al., 2008).

Nursing home (both post-acute and long-stay), assisted living, and home health care staff—that is, the long-term care workforce—may be more prepared to engage in delivery system reform because of their experience in caring for an elder population on an ongoing basis and their greater understanding of the patient/consumer's changing needs and preferences. Even this workforce, however, tends to operate in silos and, as previously described, do not have the knowledge or skills for this type of care, and the leadership in long-term care settings is often not prepared to facilitate good care coordination within and across settings.

The ACA provisions related to the development and testing of new models of coordinated and integrated care are also limited because they lack specific requirements that would ensure that the organizations participating in these programs—and receiving additional resources to do so—actually have appropriately trained and competent staff. These programs, furthermore, do not include any resources to provide additional training or technical assistance that could be used by these organizations to enhance the knowledge and skills of incumbent staff to engage in these integrated practices. Without such requirements and additional investments, it is difficult to see how better service coordination and integration can actually be achieved through the models of care legislated by the ACA.

ACA PROVISIONS ADDRESSING GERIATRIC TRAINING OF PROFESSIONAL HEALTH CARE WORKFORCE ARE INADEQUATE

The vast majority of today's workforce caring for elder Medicare beneficiaries have had no exposure to geriatric principles that include a focus on the whole person and one's informal support network, not just specific diseases, attention to the individual's functional as well as medical needs and potential for improvement, an emphasis on health promotion and wellness, recognition of the full continuum of care and service settings that are required to address individual needs over time, and an interdisciplinary, team-based approach to care delivery (Boult et al., 2010). There are only a little more than 7,000 certified geriatricians practicing in the United States today, roughly half the number presently needed. There are only 2,100 geriatric psychiatrists, fewer than half that would be necessary to provide adequate care for the current population of older adults. A number of the ACA coordinated care demonstrations rely on advanced practice nurses or social workers, most of whom have had no geriatric training. In 2008, an estimated 1.9% of advanced practice nurses were certified in gerontological nursing (U.S. Department of Health and Human Services, Health Resources and Services Administration, 2010). Fewer than 5% of social workers have identified a specialization in gerontology or geriatrics (Maiden, Horowitz, & Howe, 2010).

The lack of trained faculty is a major impediment to the development of health care professionals with the requisite knowledge, skills, and competencies to succeed in these new service delivery environments. Fewer than 1% of medical school faculty, for example, has any specialized geriatric expertise (LaMascus, Bernard, Barry, Salerno, & Weiss, 2005). Nursing schools have a much higher percentage, with 43% having full-time faculty to teach geriatrics (Bragg & Hansen, 2010–2011). The latest published data on social work education—gathered in 2000—indicated that 40% of social work schools had no faculty knowledgeable in geriatrics and gerontology (Scharlach, Damron-Rodriguez, Robinson, & Feldman, 2000).

Geriatric training is not recognized by many students or faculty as an important area of knowledge and skill development. Caring for elders as a profession often has a stigma attached to it, despite that most health care professionals encounter older adults in their practices some time during their career (Stone & Harahan, 2010). Professional schools and community colleges—where many allied health professionals receive their training—often do not encourage students to take geriatric courses or to pursue careers in geriatrics. In 2006, for example, one-third of the 442 first-year geriatric fellowship slots went unfilled. Of those positions filled, only one-third were taken by graduates of U.S. medical schools (Geriatrics Workforce Policy Studies Center, 2010). The social work literature indicates that there has been a decline in the number of master's-level social work programs providing training in gerontology and a lack of student interest in social work careers in the field of aging (Institute of Medicine, 2008).

The lack of opportunities for geriatric training is also a major challenge to preparing clinicians to provide the level of care coordination and integration required by the ACA demonstrations and models (Mezey et al., 2010–2011). The medical schools and social work programs require limited course work in geriatrics and contain little or no geriatric content in their curricula (Warshaw, Bragg, Brewer, Meganathan, & Ho, 2007; O'Neill & Barry, 2003). Social work programs have a dearth of adequate clinical placements (e.g., nursing homes or home care) where students are likely to receive good exposure to the complex care needs of chronically ill, disabled older adults (Stone & Harahan, 2010).

The ACA reforms attempt to address the educational challenges for the health professional workforce caring for older adults and younger people with disabilities. Several aspects of the ACA provisions address, to some extent, the lack of exposure to geriatric principles, opportunities for geriatric training, and trained faculty as well as the financial burdens of pursuing a career in long-term care. Perhaps the major concern is the fact that although the provisions related to geriatric training were authorized by the ACA, as of this writing, none of these programs has received an appropriation. Without adequate funding, it is not possible to expand the size and scope of these programs to new occupational categories including nursing, pharmacy, and social work.

Even if funded, the authorizations for these programs are very limited, with an average of $11 million authorized for each program or vague language authorizing "such sums as may be necessary" for the program. Given the potential increase in demand for these types of services over the next 20 years and the delivery system reform called for in the ACA, it is improbable to think that this relatively small investment (not even funded at this time) will significantly help to expand trained faculty and the workforce needed to meet these needs.

The financial burdens associated with specialized training in geriatrics pose significant challenges to the recruitment and retention of all types of professionals (Institute of Medicine, 2008). The costs associated with extra years of geriatric training do not translate into additional income, and geriatric specialists tend to earn significantly less income than specialists in other areas and often less than generalists within their own fields (Association of Directors of Geriatric Academic Programs, 2007; Health Resources and Services Administration, 2006). In part, this income disparity is due to the fact that a larger part of geriatric specialists' reimbursement tends to come from Medicare and Medicaid, where rates of reimbursement are low for the primary care codes for which these individuals bill as compared with the procedural codes typically used by other specialists. Medicare and Medicaid reimbursements do not take into account the fact that the care of frail older adults with complex needs is very time-consuming, leading to fewer patient encounters and fewer billings (Medicare Payment Advisory Commission, 2003).

Although the ACA gives bonuses to individuals who provide primary care to Medicare beneficiaries and expands both the settings and professionals eligible for this incentive, these payments will only be available for a limited time period of 5 years. Given that the major growth in the elder Medicare population will occur after this time period, it is not clear whether these bonus payments will be continued and whether this incentive will be sufficient to recruit the workforce needed to meet the demands of an elder baby boom generation. Furthermore, while geriatrics is one of the disciplines specifically identified by the ACA as eligible for the bonus payments, no resources are specifically allocated to ensure that the distribution of geriatrically trained primary care providers is sufficient to meet the needs of the elder Medicare beneficiaries.

Finally, as of this writing, the National Health Care Workforce Commission that was established by the ACA to set the nation on a path toward recruiting, training, and retaining a health care workforce has not been funded. None of the members, furthermore, has any significant background or training in caring for the elder population that could enhance the knowledge base and recommendations of this commission.

Challenges to the Development of the Direct Care Workforce and Limits of ACA

Direct care workers represent the largest component of the long-term care workforce. Numerous federal agencies, more than 35 state commissions and taskforces, many privately sponsored employers, unions and consumers, and researchers have identified the development and sustainability of a quality direct care workforce as a serious challenge in the 21st century (Institute of Medicine, 2008; Stone & Harahan, 2010). There is a widespread consensus that there are insufficient numbers of competent direct care staff to deliver long-term care services to the elder population and younger people with disabilities.

Long-term care providers and consumers face a double-edged sword. It is difficult to recruit staff due to a negative industry image, noncompetitive wages and benefits, a challenging work environment, and inadequate education and training (Stone & Dawson, 2010; Stone & Harahan, 2010). When they are recruited, staff turnover is rapid, leaving large numbers of positions vacant, putting heavy burdens on the remaining workforce, and creating further barriers to attracting and retaining a quality workforce. In 2008, the annual turnover rate among certified nurse aides was almost 43% (American Health Care Association, 2011). The comparable rate for nursing assistants employed by assisted living facilities was 29% (National Center for Assisted Living, 2011). Authors of a national synthesis of direct service worker demographics and challenges reported turnover rates for home health aides between 40% and 60% (National Direct Service Workforce Resource Center, 2008). National estimates of turnover for home care/personal care aides are not available.

Noncompetitive compensation and benefits

Direct care workers receive minimal wages and many lack health insurance coverage. In 2008, the median hourly wage of direct care workers was

$10.42, substantially below the $15.57 estimate for all workers in the United States (PHI, 2010). Forty-four percent of all direct care workers lived below 200% of the poverty level, and two in five lived in households receiving two or more public benefits such as Medicaid and food stamps (PHI, 2010). Direct care workers in long-term care settings—particularly those employed in home care—were also much less likely to have health insurance coverage than their peers in other jobs. In 2009, an estimated 28% of direct care workers were uninsured; 31% of personal care aides and 27% of nursing, psychiatric, and home health aides lacked coverage compared to 18% of all civilian workers (PHI, 2011). There are, furthermore, large disparities across settings. The hospital setting has the lowest percentage of direct care workers without health insurance (14%) compared to the home health services industry (37%) and nursing homes and residential care facilities (26%) (PHI, 2011).

CHALLENGING WORK ENVIRONMENT

Workforce environments typically do not support frontline supervisors and direct care workers, starting with a hierarchical chain of command structure that discourages involvement of lower-level staff in care planning and ongoing decision making. Not surprisingly, nursing assistants and home health/home care aides do not feel that their jobs are respected, a perception that contributes to job dissatisfaction and high turnover rates (Bishop et al., 2008; Bowers, Esmond, & Jacobson, 2003; Wiener, Squillace, Anderson, & Khatusky, 2009). Other workforce challenges include inflexible work flow and job design, ethnic and racial tensions due to cultural diversity of staff and consumers in long-term care settings, and a paucity of career advancement opportunities (Wiener et al., 2009; Castle & Engberg, 2006).

Caring for older adults can be physically taxing. Direct care staff in nursing homes has one of the highest rates of workplace injury among all occupations. In 2009, the rate of nonfatal occupational injury and illness involving days away from work was 456 incidents per 10,000 workers among nursing aides, orderlies, and attendants (Bureau of Labor Statistics, 2010).

INADEQUATE EDUCATION AND TRAINING

The preparation of potential candidates for direct care positions and ongoing training for those working in the field are out of sync with the realities of the demand for long-term care and its practice. Studies have found that the perception of adequate preparation and training (both initial and in-service) on the part of nursing assistants is highly correlated with job satisfaction, which in turn is associated with direct care worker turnover and quality of care outcomes (Sengupta, Harris-Kojetin, & Ejaz, 2010). Nevertheless, the strategies employed by regulators and educators to prepare and certify this workforce and to assure that personnel are able to keep pace with changes in the clinical knowledge base and new technologies are inadequate. To become a Medicare- or Medicaid-certified home health aide, federal law requires less than 2 weeks of training and passing a competency exam. Federal continuing education requirements for home health aides are minimal, and content is left to states and providers. The regulation of other direct care workers, including those who work in assisted living and personal care and home care agencies, is determined by the states. Typically, staff in these settings receives little or no training (Seavey, 2007). There are also relatively few standards or competencies specific to long-term care. There is, furthermore, a huge shortfall of personnel who are competent and committed to educating and preparing direct care workers for long-term care careers. This translates into a dearth of people—both current and in the pipeline—who are adequately trained and educated to assume increasingly complex jobs across the continuum of care.

This inadequacy of investment in education and training is compounded by the complexities of chronically disabled elder individuals, the current push towards new models of care, and the prevailing trend toward more sophisticated technology. Direct care workers require formal training and ongoing education for improving their knowledge and skills to respond to new philosophies and models. Movements such as culture change, which transform the nursing home environment, will become more widely adopted through efforts such as ACA (Weiner & Ronch, 2003; Miller et al., 2010).

The increasingly complex physical and mental health needs of community-dwelling chronically disabled elder individuals call for more highly skilled direct care workers trained in areas such as medication management, dementia care, and palliative care. As service integration across settings becomes more widespread with implementation of the ACA coordinated care provisions, these frontline staff may also be incorporated into clinical teams. Empowerment of direct care workers and effective supervision are strategies to prepare the frontline staff. Nurse delegation, which expands home care aides' scope of practice and allows nurses to delegate more complex tasks, can empower direct care workers, increase their responsibility, and reduce program costs (Reinhard, 2011). A number of studies have found that coaching and education are much more successful strategies for effective supervision than traditional "command and control" strategies (Stone, 2007). Unfortunately, the literature also underscores the fact that nurse managers typically are not trained in how effectively to supervise direct care workers. The growth in publicly funded consumer-directed programs that give the consumer the resources and the authority to hire and fire their workers—including their own family members—raises serious workforce issues. These include the magnitude and scope of training that should be required and the roles and responsibilities that consumers can or must assume when they become employers (Foster, Schmitz, & Kemper, 2007).

ACA PROVISIONS ADDRESSING RECRUITMENT AND RETENTION OF DIRECT CARE WORKERS

The ACA is the first federal legislative effort specifically to address the development of the direct care workforce. This represents a major step forward in the acknowledgment of the pivotal role these workers play in delivering care and the need to strengthen this workforce. However, the provisions do not adequately address many of the barriers to recruiting and retaining these workers, including noncompetitive compensation and benefits (with the exception of universal health insurance coverage) and an unsatisfactory work environment. The ACA is limited in its efforts to focus on the education and training of these workers as well.

When the ACA takes full effect in 2014, health insurance coverage through Medicaid could be extended to many uninsured direct care workers with and without children. Targeted outreach, however, will be especially important for enrolling workers employed in home care settings, since they lack a conventional workplace where standard outreach materials might reach them (PHI, 2011). The prospect of state-based insurance exchanges offering access to affordable insurance for small businesses and to individuals not covered by their employers is also a promising development. At the same time, over the next 2 years, employers and state Medicaid programs will need to examine the cost of employer-sponsored insurance and the viability of building the cost of health coverage into reimbursement rates that elder care providers receive in order for these employers to comply with the new law.

Despite the significance of the ACA in its recognition of paraprofessionals, the provisions related to direct care workers are limited in terms of addressing both the supply and quality of these individuals. The ACA's emphasis on shifting long-term care resources from institutional settings to home- and community-based care has the potential to increase significantly the demand for direct care workers—particularly home health, home care, and personal care aides. The inadequate supply of a community-based workforce has recently been identified as one of the key obstacles to the success of the Money Follows the Person program in transitioning nursing home residents to community-based settings (O'Malley Watts, 2011). If that program were to expand in response to the ACA incentives, concerns about the supply of workers would only escalate. Furthermore, if the Community Living Assistance Services and Supports (CLASS) voluntary insurance program had been implemented, many middle class older adults (as well as younger people with disabilities) would have had the resources to purchase home care, placing additional demands on the supply of workers.

Serious questions are currently being raised about the extent to which these elements of the ACA will go into effect, particularly in light of the current economic climate. The Secretary of the Department of Health and Human Services, for example, recently halted efforts to implement the CLASS insurance program, and Congressional concerns about the solvency of CLASS have made this program a target for repeal. Failure to implement CLASS obviates, to a certain extent, the need for an expanded home- and community-based direct care workforce, at least in the short term. The need to expand this workforce will further be obviated if the ACA's home- and community-based service provisions prove unsuccessful in stimulating state action in this area, particularly in light of challenges posed by the prevailing fiscal environment.

Nevertheless, the need to address the recruitment and retention issues described above will remain a challenge. Although the legislation authorized over $65 million over a 4-year period to provide grants and incentives for enhancing recruitment and retention of direct care staff, the language is vague and the funds have yet to be appropriated. The deliberations of the Personal Care Attendants Workforce Advisory Panel, charged with examining and advising the Secretary of Department of Health and Human Services and Congress on the current and future adequacy of the number of home care and personal care aides, have stalled in light of the uncertainties surrounding the implementation of the CLASS Act provisions and Medicaid home- and community-based care expansions.

The incentives provided to states to expand their criminal background check efforts could actually reduce the pool of candidates for these jobs. Given the fact that individuals seeking low-wage jobs are more likely to have engaged in some type of criminal activity than those pursuing higher-wage jobs, expanded criminal background checks could exclude individuals who would otherwise be hired in the long-term care sector. The Department of Health and Human Services Office of the Inspector General is currently conducting an evaluation of this initiative to assess the effects of the program on the supply of workers and employer challenges to recruitment.

The ACA workforce provisions targeted to the direct care workforce are very limited in terms of addressing the orientation and in-service training required to ensure that these workers have the knowledge and skills to deliver quality services in the range of long-term care settings. Most of the training opportunities for direct care workers have been authorized but not appropriated. The addition of dementia and elder abuse prevention training to the minimum national training requirements for certified nursing assistants is a welcomed change. The failure of the ACA, however, to increase the minimum number of required hours means that these content areas will have to be incorporated into an already packed curriculum.

The most promising effort in this area is the state-based demonstration, currently being administered by the Health Resources and Services Administration, that will help the field understand the feasibility of developing and implementing standardized core competencies for home care/personal care aides at the state level and how worker training for these caregivers might be integrated into the development of quality home- and community-based service systems. It is the first national initiative to recognize the need for core competencies and competency-based training to prepare individuals who will be employed directly by consumers through the self-directed options expanded in the ACA.

This demonstration program, however, is limited to six states and the evaluation of this program is in its first phase. Widespread dissemination of the core competencies developed through the program and the results of the impact evaluation (should they be positive) will be required if the effort is to go beyond the research stage. Although staff in the Health Resources and Services Administration has primary responsibility for most of the workforce initiatives included in the ACA, this is the only activity specifically related to the direct care workforce. Historically, the agency has not focused any attention on this workforce, has little knowledge or staff capacity in this area, and has little communication with other agencies that influence the demand for and supply of these workers. The ability of this agency, therefore, to disseminate the findings through various channels (including the Centers for Medicare and Medicaid Services, which is responsible for the Medicaid home- and community-based service programs that employ direct care workers) is questionable.

The pot of money authorized for grants to enhance recruitment and retention of direct care workers includes some references to career ladders and wage/benefit increases as well as improving management practices but, as noted above, no funds have been appropriated for these grants. Furthermore, it is difficult to see how states or employers could engage in these types of activities within the current economic climate, where they have few resources to invest in such efforts. The culture change demonstration provides opportunities for nursing homes to test new organizational structures within the nursing home setting that support self-managed work teams in resident households and the use of universal frontline workers who are responsible for all of the tasks within a household such as personal care, cooking, laundry, recreation, and communication with nursing staff (Weiner & Ronch, 2003; Miller et al., 2010). This project will help identify best practices for providers who have the resources and choose to create small houses or other household models. The findings, however, will need to be disseminated to and used by the larger group of nursing home providers that have not embraced culture change to improve the working conditions of their direct care workers.

CONCLUSION

The ACA is groundbreaking legislation in its explicit recognition of the need for a quality workforce within the context of health care reform, its attention to geriatric training and expanding the professional pipeline trained in this area, and its special focus on direct care workers. These provisions, however, are seriously limited in terms of a lack of dedicated funding and their ability to increase significantly the number of competent professionals and direct care workers who can effectively meet the current demand, let alone the additional demands associated with delivery system reforms and the aging of the population over the next 20 years. Many of the demonstration provisions in the ACA simply assume that participating organizations have the workforce capacity to implement successfully the new models being evaluated. Unfortunately, these payment and delivery system reforms may be doomed to failure without the appropriate investment in education, ongoing training, and adequate compensation to attract and retain this workforce.

REFERENCES

Abrams, M., Nuzum, R., Mika, S., & Lawlor, G. (2011). *How the Affordable Care Act will strengthen primary care and benefit patients, providers and payers.* The Commonwealth Fund, Publication 1466, Volume 1.

Association of Directors of Geriatric Academic Programs. (2007). Fellows in geriatric medicine and geriatric psychiatry programs. *Training & Practice Update, 5*(2), 1–7.

American Health Care Association. (2011). *Report of findings: Nursing facility staffing survey 2010.* Retrieved from http://www.ahcancal.org/research_data/staffing/Documents/REPORT%20OF%20FINDINGS%20NURSING%20FACILITY%20STAFFING%20SURVEY%202010.pdf

Bishop, C. E., Weinberg, D. B., Leutz, W., Dossa, A., Pfefferle, S. G., & Zincavage, R. M. (2008). Nursing assistants' job commitment: Effect of nursing home organizational factors and impact on resident well-being. *The Gerontologist, 48*(Special Issue 1), 36–45.

Boult, C., Christmas, C., Durso, S. C., Leff, B., Boult, L. B., & Fried, L. P. (2008). Perspective: Transforming chronic care for older persons. *Academic Medicine, 83*(7), 627–631.

Bowers, B. J., Esmond, S., & Jacobson, N. (2003). Turnover reinterpreted: CNAs talk about why they leave. *Journal of Gerontological Nursing, 29*(3), 36–43.

Bragg, E., & Hansen, J. C. (2010–2011). A revelation of numbers: Will America's eldercare workforce be ready to care for an aging America? *Generations, 34*(4), 11–19.

Bureau of Labor Statistics. (2010). *Nonfatal occupational injuries and illnesses requiring days away from work, 2009.* Retrieved from http://www.bls.gov/news.release/archives/osh2_11092010.pdf

Castle, G. C., & Engberg, J. (2006). Organizational characteristics associated with staff turnover in nursing homes. *Gerontologist, 46*(1), 62–73.

Counsell, S. R., Callahan, C. M., Clark, D. O., Tu, W., Buttar, A. B., Stump, T. E., & Ricketts, G. D. (2007). Geriatric care management for low-income seniors. *Journal of the American Medical Association, 298*(22), 2623–2633.

Fisher, E. S., Staiger, D. O., Bynum, J., & Gottlieb, D. J. (2007). Creating accountable care organizations: The extended hospital medical staff. *Health Affairs, 26*(1), w44–w57.

Foster, L., Schmitz, R., & Kemper, P. (2007). *The effects of PACE on Medicare and Medicaid expenditures. Report to CMS*. Princeton, NJ: Mathematica Policy Research Inc.

Geriatrics Workforce Policy Studies Center. (2010). *Documenting the development of geriatric medicine*. Retrieved from http://www.adgapstudy.uc.edu/faq.cfm

Health Resources and Services Administration. (2006). *The registered nurse population: Findings from the March 2004 National Sample Survey of Registered Nurses*. Washington, DC: Health Resources and Services Administration.

Institute of Medicine. (2008). *Retooling for an aging America: Building the health care workforce*. Washington, DC: National Academies Press.

Justice, D. (2010). *Long-term services and supports and chronic care coordination: Policy advances enacted by the Patient Protection and Affordable Care Act*. National Academy for State Health Policy. Retrieved from http://www.nashp.org/node/1903

LaMascus, A. M., Bernard, M. A., Barry, P., Salerno, J., & Weiss, J. (2005). Bridging the workforce gap for our aging society: How to increase and improve knowledge and training. Report of an expert panel. *Journal of the American Geriatrics Society, 53*(2), 343–347.

Maiden, R. J., Horowitz, B. P., & Howe, J. L. (2010). Workforce training and education gaps in gerontology and geriatrics: What we found in New York State. *Gerontology and Geriatrics Education, 31*(4), 328–348.

McClellan, M., McKethan, A. N., Lewis, J. L., Roski, J., & Fisher, E. S. (2010). A national strategy to put accountable care into practice. *Health Affairs, 19*(5), 982–990.

Medicare Payment Advisory Commission. (2003). *Impact of the resident caps on the supply of geriatricians*. Washington, DC: Medicare Payment Advisory Commission.

Mezey, M., Mitty, E., Cortes, T., Burger, S., Clark, E., & McCallion, P. (2010–2011). A competency-based approach to educating and training the eldercare workforce. *Generations, 34*(4), 53–60.

Miller, S. C., Miller, E. A., Jung, H. Y., Sterns, S., Clark, M. A., & Mor, V. (2010). Nursing home organizational change: The "culture change" movement as viewed by long-term care specialists. *Medical Care Research and Review, 64*(4 Suppl.), 65S–81S.

National Center for Assisted Living. (2011). *Findings for the NCAL 2010 assisted living staff vacancy, retention and turnover survey*. Retrieved from http://www.ahcancal.org/ncal/resources/Documents/2010%20VRT%20Report-Final.pdf

National Direct Service Workforce Resource Center. (2008). *A synthesis of direct service workforce demographics and challenges across intellectual/developmental disabilities, aging, physical disabilities, and behavioral health*. Retrieved from http://rtc.umn.edu/docs/Cross-DisabilitySynthesisWhitePaperFinal.pdf

O'Malley Watts, M. (2011). *Money Follows the Person: A 2010 snapshot, February 2011*. Retrieved from http://www.kff.org/medicaid/upload/8142.pdf

O'Neill, G., & Barry, P. P. (2003). Training physicians in geriatric care: Responding to critical need. *Public Policy and Aging Report, 13*(2), 17–21.

PHI. (2010). *Who are the direct care workers? February 2010 update. Facts 3*. Retrieved from http://www.directcareclearinghouse.org/download/NCDCW%20Fact%20Sheet-1.pdf

PHI. (2011). *Health care coverage for direct care workers: 2009 data update. Facts 4*. Issue Brief supported by a grant from the SCAN Foundation.

Reinhard, S. C. (2011). A case for nurse-delegation explores a new frontier in consumer-directed patient care. *Generations, 34*(4), 75–81. Retrieved from http://www.cshp.rutgers.edu/Downloads/320.pdf

Scharlach, A., Damron-Rodriguez, J., Robinson, B., & Feldman, R. (2000). Educating social workers for an aging society: A vision for the 21st century. *Journal of Social Work Education, 36*(3), 521–538.

Seavey, D. (2007). *Written statement of Dorie Seavey, Ph.D*. Testimony before the House Committee on Education and Labor, Subcommittee on Workforce Protections, Washington, DC. October 25.

Sengupta, M., Harris-Kojetin, L. D., & Ejaz, F. K. (2010). A national overview of the training received by certified nursing assistants in U.S. nursing homes. *Gerontology and Geriatric Education, 31*(3), 201–219.

Stone, R. (2007). Introduction. *Gerontology and Geriatrics Education, 28*(2), 5–16.

Stone, R. I., & Dawson, S. (2008). The origins of better jobs better care. *The Gerontologist, 48*(Special Issue), 5–13.

Stone, R. I., & Harahan, M. F. (2010). Improving the long-term care workforce serving older adults. *Health Affairs, 29*(1), 109–115.

U.S. Department of Health and Human Services, Health Resources and Services Administration. (2010). *The registered nurse population: Findings from the 2008 National Sample Survey of Registered Nurses*. Retrieved from http://bhpr.hrsa.gov/healthworkforce/rnsurvey2008.html

Warhsaw, G. A., Bragg, E. J., Brewer, D. E., Meganathan, K., & Ho, M. (2007). The development of academic geriatric medicine: Progress toward preparing the nation's physicians to care for an aging population. *Journal of the American Geriatrics Society, 55*, 2075–2082.

Weiner, A. S., & Ronch, J .L. (Eds.). (2003). *Culture change in long-term care*. New York, NY: Haworth Social Work Practice Press.

Wiener, J., Squillace, M., Anderson, W., & Khatusky, G. (2009). Why do they stay? Job tenure among certified nursing assistants in nursing homes. *The Gerontologist, 49*(2), 198–210.

Nursing Homes and the Affordable Care Act: A Cease Fire in the Ongoing Struggle Over Quality Reform

CATHERINE HAWES, PhD

Regents Professor Department of Health Policy and Management, School of Rural Public Health, Texas A&M Health Science Center, College Station, Texas, USA

DARCY M. MOUDOUNI, PhD

Assistant Research Scientist Department of Health Policy and Management, School of Rural Public Health, Texas A&M Health Science Center, College Station, Texas, USA

RACHEL B. EDWARDS, BA

Doctoral Student Department of Health Policy and Management, School of Rural Public Health, Texas A&M Health Science Center, College Station, Texas, USA

CHARLES D. PHILLIPS, PhD, MPH

Regents Professor, Department of Health Policy and Management, School of Rural Public Health, Texas A&M Health Science Center, College Station, Texas, USA

Most provisions in the Affordable Care Act that affect nursing homes originated in two earlier attempts at reform, both of which failed multiple times in prior Congressional sessions: the Elder Justice Act and the Nursing Home Transparency and Improvement Act. Both of these earlier efforts focused on improving quality and reducing elder abuse in nursing homes by strengthening oversight and enforcement penalties, expanding staff training, and increasing the information on nursing home quality available to consumers and regulators. Each bill addressed problems that were serious, widespread, and had persisted for years, but each failed to pass on its own. The Affordable Care Act, with its own momentum, became the vehicle for their passage. However, the reasons the bills failed in these earlier efforts suggest implementation challenges now that they have ridden into law on the coattails of the more general effort to reform the health care sector.

INTRODUCTION

In 2010, Congress passed and President Obama signed into law the Patient Protection and Affordable Care Act (ACA) of 2010 (Pub. L. No. 111-148), as amended by the Health Care and Education Reconciliation Act of 2010 (Pub L. No. 111-152). This act's primary nursing home (NH) provisions were originally parts of bills introduced previously in multiple sessions of Congress that languished and died in committees or subcommittees, never garnering sufficient attention or support to pass on their own. However, when folded into the ACA, they were resuscitated—at least in terms of becoming law. How these provisions will fare in terms of funding and implementation in the current political and fiscal climates remains to be seen.

The first bill that failed to pass was known as the Elder Justice Act (EJA), the second as the NH Transparency and Improvement Act. As stand-alone bills, each addressed widespread and serious problems that had persisted for years. The EJA was first introduced in the 107th Congress in 2002 and in each successive Congress—the 108th, 109th, and 110th—and failed to pass. The NH Transparency and Improvement Act was introduced in the Senate and House in the 110th and again in the Senate in the 111th Congress but never made it out of the committees or subcommittees to which they were assigned.

The reality is that neither the EJA nor the NH Transparency and Improvement Act was likely to become law without being folded into the ACA. The EJA engendered little opposition but also had an inadequate sense of urgency to secure passage. The NH Transparency and Improvement Act, however, generated considerable opposition from the NH industry, containing as it did elements that the industry had fought for decades. Thus, the provisions of the ACA affecting NHs were not new ideas but previously stalled reforms.

To understand the elements of the ACA related to NHs, we consider the background and legislative history of both the EJA and the NH Transparency and Improvement Act. This includes discussion of the politics surrounding the bills, since the factors contributing to their failure are suggestive of their likely fate during implementation of the ACA. We also discuss the ACA provisions and their likely impact, given the dynamics of the EJA and NH Transparency and Improvement Act and prior NH reforms.

BACKGROUND ON THE EJA

A 2009 national survey estimated that 14.1% of noninstitutionalized older adults had experienced some form of elder abuse in the past 12 months, a figure that would be higher if the cognitively impaired and people in residential long-term care (LTC) settings had not been excluded from the study (Acierno et al., 2010). Prior to 2002, however, the topic was rarely raised in Congress, the White House, or executive agencies, relatively anemic exceptions notwithstanding, including meager federal funding for adult protective services (Mixson, 2010; Teaster, Wangmo, & Anetzberger, 2010; United States Senate Special Committee on Aging, 2011; U.S. Government Accountability Office [GAO], 2011). Furthermore, despite congressional hearings and reports and studies detailing the nature of elder abuse and neglect (Bonnie & Wallace, 2002; United States House Select Committee on Aging, Subcommittee on Health and Long-Term Care, 1985, 1990, 1991), only one House bill related to the identification and treatment of elder abuse was introduced during the 1980s, and it was not enacted.

NH reform included in the Omnibus Budget Reconciliation Act of 1987 (OBRA '87) (Pub L. 100-203) addressed elder abuse but only in NHs. It specified that residents were to be free of abuse, neglect, and exploitation and mandated actions by both NHs and the states that were designed to prevent elder abuse in nursing facilities. However, it left elder mistreatment in other settings unaddressed, and the only federal agency touched by the law was the Center for Medicare and Medicaid Services (CMS). It was not until the 2002 publication of a comprehensive report by the National Research Council (NRC), *Elder Mistreatment: Abuse, Neglect, and Exploitation in an Aging America* (Bonnie & Wallace, 2002), that sufficient momentum for the development of more comprehensive legislation arrived.

The findings of the NRC report were reinforced by another documenting widespread NH citations for abuse in a report by Representative Waxman's Investigations Division of the Committee on Government Reform (United States House Committee on Government Reform, Special Investigations Division, 2001), a spate of newspaper series on elder abuse, growing public concern, and testimony at a 2002 hearing on elder abuse held by the U.S. Senate Finance Committee. The first result was S. 2933, the EJA, sponsored by Senator John Breaux (D-LA), with 19 bipartisan cosponsors. S. 2933 was introduced on September 12, 2002, and immediately referred to the Committee on Finance, where it quietly expired since practically no time was left for hearings or votes in the 107th Congress.

This pattern of bipartisan support continued, even after Senator Breaux left the Senate and Senator Orrin Hatch (R-UT) became the EJA's sponsor. The same was true in the House, with Democrat Rahm Emanuel alternating sponsorship with Republican Peter King in the 108th, 109th, 110th, and 111th Congresses. For each Congress, from the 107th in 2001–2002 to the 111th in 2009–2010, the bills either died in committee/subcommittee or, if placed on the Senate Legislative Calendar, never came up for a vote. Thus, despite bipartisan Congressional support in the House and Senate, relatively little controversy or opposition, a fairly modest fiscal impact, and a devoted (if not well-funded) coalition of advocates, the EJA continued to languish.

It seems incomprehensible that a bill with fairly widespread bipartisan support and relatively minor opposition continued to fail for so long. One contributing factor may have been more general NH industry opposition to increased government oversight, including EJA requirements that facilities report criminal abuse to law enforcement and the application of fines (civil monetary penalties [CMPs]) for failing to do so (Schulte, 2008). On the other hand, there was a 699-member Elder Justice Coalition that steadfastly supported the EJA throughout its history. The coalition was composed of a variety of organizations and individuals and included the National Committee for the Prevention of Elder Abuse and the National Adult Protective Services Association, advocacy groups for LTC residents (e.g., the Consumer Voice for Quality Long-Term Care, originally the National Citizens Coalition for Nursing Home Reform), and other groups advocating more broadly for older persons, such as AARP and the Gray Panthers, as well as other well-connected organizations, such as the Family Research Council and Alzheimer's Association.

Lindberg, Sabatino, and Blancato (2011) revealed that the proximate reasons for the Act's failure varied from session to session. Sometimes it was the self-interested machinations of an individual senator. For example, in one session, an individual senator prevented a floor vote as part of a strategy to force some of the bills' cosponsors to support a different piece of legislation. In the House, committee jurisdiction complicated the issue. The bill was usually referred to four committees—Ways and Means, Judiciary, Energy and Commerce, and Education and Labor—since the EJA had provisions that fell under the auspices of each. This made agreement difficult, resulting in the bill's death in one of those committees. Also, Bush Administration officials opposed the bill at various times, arguing that existing programs in the Administration on Aging, the Department of Justice, and CMS were sufficient to address the elder abuse issue.

It is also true that the EJA got lost among the thousands of bills introduced in Congress each year, only a small fraction of which were enacted: 5.5%, on average, over the course of the last decade and 3.3% in the 110th Congress (2007–2008). These percentages of bills passed are the lowest since 1976, down from 15% to 20% in earlier decades (Singer, 2008). Most bills died in committee or subcommittee, with no major action taken, as was the case with the EJA. Bills need tremendous momentum to escape a quiet death in committees. The EJA, while not attracting significant opposition, was never a priority for the leadership of either party and did not generate sufficient attention in the media and among the public to pressure Congress to move it ahead on the policy agenda. Nonetheless, the EJA was kept alive, albeit on life support, for 8 years by the clear need for action in this area, its bipartisan support in Congress, and ongoing advocacy by citizen groups.

BACKGROUND ON THE NH TRANSPARENCY AND IMPROVEMENT ACT

The NH Transparency Acts of 2008 and 2009 were, in part, the products of more than a decade of investigations and hearings on continuing quality problems and regulatory failures despite comprehensive reforms included in OBRA '87. OBRA '87 mandated improvements in the standards governing facilities, the inspection or survey process intended to determine facilities' compliance with standards, and enforcement mechanisms. Early evaluations of the OBRA '87 reforms, which focused largely on the effect of the new standards, found significant improvements in quality of care and quality of life (Hawes et al., 1997; Mor et al., 1997; Phillips et al. 1997). However, several factors attenuated OBRA '87's impact over time as the regulations became more weakly enforced (Kumar, Norton, & Encinosa, 2006).

First, the standards failed to mandate adequate staffing levels and training requirements. Second, the Clinton Administration's focus on reducing the deficit led to significant cutbacks in federal support for the inspection processes. Third, at the NH industry's behest, there was a steady reduction in enforcement remedies and processes (Edelman, 1997–1998). Fourth, with the support of both consumers and the industry—and in conjunction with the rising antiregulatory attitude in Washington—there was a growing focus on quality improvement and "culture change," supplanting an emphasis on strong regulation (Edelman, 1997–1998; Gagel, 1995).

In the decade preceding the introduction of the NH Transparency Acts, the U.S. GAO and Department of Health and Human Services Office of Inspector General issued numerous reports on NH quality and safety (United States Department of Health and Human Services, Office of Inspector General, 2006; U.S. GAO, 1999, 2003, 2005, 2007, 2008, 2009). These identified serious and widespread problems with NH regulation. Prominent findings included failure of the federally mandated inspections of NHs to detect serious problems, lack of timely surveys, inadequate investigation and resolution of complaints, and failure to use enforcement remedies effectively. In addition, GAO studies found the existence of "repeat offenders," NHs that persistently provided seriously substandard care. It was also found

THE AFFORDABLE CARE ACT

that CMS and the state agencies had insufficient resources to implement all of the needed quality improvement initiatives.

Based on their joint work on NH quality, Senators Grassley (R-IA) and Kohl (D-WI) authored the NH Transparency and Improvement Act of 2008 (S. 2641). This bill focused on strengthening regulation, particularly by increasing CMPs for serious quality problems or repeat offenses, improving the complaint resolution processes, improving the monitoring of multifacility NH "chains," and enhancing consumer information related to NH quality, such as inspection results, the size of a facility's staff, and facility ownership information. A similar bill, introduced in the House (H.R. 7128) by Democratic Representatives Stark (CA-13) and Schakowsky (IL-9), contained many of the same provisions but also specified more demanding disclosure requirements for NHs owned by large private equity firms and on facilities that had a corporate structure that limited their liability in cases of neglect/malpractice and disguised multifacility ownership by common parties. These and a subsequent Senate version (S. 647) died in committee/subcommittee during the 110th and 111th Congress.

The legislation attracted both supporters and opponents. Twenty unique organizations filed reports on their lobbying activities on the three bills. The supporters of the legislation included a mix of well-known national organizations with paid lobbyists and small, nonprofit consumer groups without paid lobbyists. Some, such as the National Consumer Voice for Quality Long-Term Care, spoke with members and Congressional staff about the need for the bills; others, such as AARP, Service Employees International Union, and Families USA, were formally registered as lobbying on the NH Transparency Acts.

The opponents were smaller in number but politically more powerful because they had well-funded lobbying organizations and political action committees that focused almost all of their attention on NH payment and regulation. The two main opponents were the American Health Care Organization (AHCA), representing for-profit providers, and The Alliance for Quality Nursing Home Care (AQNHC), representing multifacility NH "chains." They were joined by individual NH chains and private equity and real estate investment management firms that owned facilities. The American Association of Homes and Services for the Aging (AAHSA; now LeadingAge), representing nonprofit providers, was also active but took a different stance on most provisions than AHCA and AQNHC.

The most contentious provision was that the NH Transparency and Improvement Act would have increased the penalties that CMS and the states could impose on NHs for violations of standards, with a penalty of up to $100,000 for a deficiency resulting in death, fines of $3,000 to $25,000 for deficiencies that caused actual harm or placed a resident in immediate jeopardy of harm, and fines of not more than $3,000 for other deficiencies. Consumer advocates strongly supported this, arguing that the existing low fines were treated by some facilities as a cost of doing business and were frequently so low that they have failed to secure compliance by NHs that had a pattern of repeated noncompliance (U.S. GAO, 2007). Studies have consistently shown that regulatory agencies seldom impose significant penalties, with fines imposed often being too low given the nature of the deficiencies (Reichard, 2008; U.S. GAO, 2007). Supporters thus strongly supported increasing penalties so that they might become a more meaningful deterrent (Pear, 2008).

NH representatives opposed the increase in CMPs (Pear, 2008; Schulte, 2008). The industry has traditionally argued against aggressive enforcement, favoring "less punitive" initiatives such as consultation on quality improvement or culture change initiatives (Edelman, 1997–1998; Pear, 2008). The proprietary industry also opposed the requirement for greater reporting on transparency of ownership and staffing information. The intention of these provisions was to enable state and federal regulators and consumers to identify all persons and entities with a significant ownership stake or who were affiliated or related parties, such as firms with management contracts or that own and lease the real estate. These provisions were a product of changes in the NH industry over the preceding decade that made it more difficult to identify NHs that had common underlying ownership and were, in reality, part of a NH chain. This included reorganization of some facilities as limited liability companies, which do not identify themselves as part of a group of facilities with a common set of owners, and the acquisition of several NH chains from publicly traded companies by private equity firms (Duhigg, 2007). Both of these changes made it difficult for consumers and regulators to identify the individuals or corporations that controlled an NH and, therefore, to hold them accountable and to seek resolution when quality problems occurred (Reichard, 2008). Research also indicated a rise in deficiencies among chains being taken over by private equity firms (Duhigg, 2007; Harrington, Olney, Carrillo, & Kang, 2011).

As a result of these problems, representatives of state and federal agencies responsible for enforcement of Medicare and Medicaid fraud and elder abuse testified in favor of the proposed legislation, joining the consumer groups who supported the NH Transparency and Improvement Act (Pear, 2008; Reichard, 2008). In addition, AAHSA supported the enhanced reporting of ownership and finances, including spending on direct care staff. In part, this was because they already provided this information to qualify with the IRS for not-for-profit tax status. In addition, AAHSA represents NHs that traditionally have higher staffing levels, so reporting those data to the public would be a plus for those facilities. There was also concern that care for vulnerable people not be treated as a "commodities business" by private equity firms where the primary goal is to maximize value for investors through diversified portfolios rather than concentrating on providing quality care to residents (Reichard, 2008; Schulte, 2008).

In contrast, the AHCA and others representing NH chains and private equity firms argued that new organizational structures such as these were necessary to shield the industry from liability, that is, from the "enterprising attorneys" who sued them (Schulte, 2008). They also repeated their common argument that the increased "paperwork burden" of the enhanced reporting on ownership, finances, and staffing required by the act would take staff time away from providing care and that more transparency was not a solution but could, in other words, lead to worse quality of care (Schulte, 2008).

Ultimately, strong opposition from the for-profit sector of the NH industry, including the private equity and real estate holding companies, affected the fate of the NH Transparency and Improvement Act, as did timing of the bills in an election year in 2008 and during the initial debates over health care reform in 2009 during which other concerns took precedence. Thus, the heavier CMPs found in the 2008 version of the NH Transparency and Improvement Act were dropped from the 2009 version, while neither version of the bill achieved passage. However, with the election of President Obama and the introduction of bills that eventually became the ACA, political serendipity began to favor the EJA and the NH Transparency and Improvement Act of 2009.

PROVISIONS OF THE ACA AFFECTING NHs

Early during the first session it became clear that the EJA would not pass the 111th Congress on its own (Lindberg et al., 2011). The same was true of the NH Transparency and Improvement Act. The only possibility was to incorporate both into the final version of the health care reform bill. On November 7, 2009, the House voted 220 to 215 in favor of the Affordable Health Care for America Act. The bill did not include any of the provisions included in the EJA and NH Transparency and Improvement Act bills. In the Senate, as the health care reform debate progressed, EJA and NH Transparency and Improvement Act supporters concluded that a bipartisan bill would not emerge from the efforts of the "Gang of Six" on the Senate Finance Committee (Oberlander, 2010). As a result, it fell to members of the Democratic leadership and Senators Lincoln (D-AR) and Kohl (D-WI) to negotiate for inclusion of the EJA and NH Transparency and Improvement Act provisions, respectively, in the final Senate bill.

When the Obama Administration finally released its priorities for health care reform, it included the EJA, and both the EJA and NH Transparency and Improvement Act were subsequently incorporated into the ACA passed by the Senate on December 24, 2009, by a vote of 60–39, with all the Democrats and two Independents voting for and all 39 Republicans voting against. On March 21, 2010, the Senate version passed the House by a vote of 219 to

212, with all 178 Republicans and 34 Democrats voting against. It was signed into law by President Obama on March 23, 2010.

There are many provisions in the ACA that will affect long term services and supports, and some, such as efforts to rebalance the LTC system, may indirectly affect NHs. Most, though not all, provisions directly affecting NHs were part of the EJA or NH Transparency and Improvement Act. The general goals were to improve quality and reduce abuse and neglect of residents through four basic mechanisms: increasing transparency of information; enhancing facility accountability and capacity; improving the quality and skills of staff; and strengthening quality assurance mechanisms (Center for Medicare Advocacy, 2010).

Transparency and Consumer Information

The general goal of the transparency provisions was to make relevant information accessible to the public, including consumers, their advocates, and the regulators responsible for ensuring residents' safety and the quality of their care. These provisions fit with the general goal of increasing transparency throughout the health care system and strengthening consumer information systems. In short, NHs must report more information on direct and indirect controlling interests in the operation and management of the facility, including officers, directors, shareholders, partners, and trustees who have ownership interests, managerial control, provide management services or lease or sublease real property. They must also report how they allocate their spending across key categories, including direct care; indirect care, such as dietary services and housekeeping; administrative expenses; and capital assets, presumably including rents or lease payments. Data on staffing must be reported to CMS as well, based on auditable information, such as payroll data, and must include hours of care per resident/day for each category of direct care worker, wages and benefits, and information on staff turnover, as well as information about resident census and the intensity of resident needs (case mix) so that the staffing levels can be evaluated in terms of adequacy.

The transparency provisions expand the information on each facility that will be included on or linked to CMS's Nursing Home Compare Web site, including staffing levels and turnover; links to state Web sites that have survey reports and a facility's plan to correct deficiencies; summary information on the number, type, severity, and outcome of substantiated complaints; and the number of criminal violations by the facility or its employees. In addition, there will be a consumer rights information page on the Web site that helps consumers interpret the information on Nursing Home Compare and links to LTC ombudsmen programs in the states. The GAO is also to study CMS's 5-Star Rating System, which provides public rating of facilities based on their staffing, deficiencies, and Minimum Data Set–based quality indicators. The GAO study will describe how the system is being implemented and how the system can be improved.

Facility Accountability and Quality Improvement

The ACA mandates several actions that NHs must implement as part of quality improvement and accountability. NHs are required to create and implement a compliance and ethics program aimed at preventing and detecting criminal, civil, and administrative violations and an internal quality assurance and performance improvement program to develop best practices to meet standards. They must also give at least 60 days' notice of voluntary closure and must have a transfer and relocation plan for residents approved by the state. A facility that does not comply may be subject to a CMP of up to $100,000 and be excluded from participation in Medicare and Medicaid. The ACA provides for demonstration programs to test best practices for achieving culture change in facilities and for using information technology to improve resident care as well.

Two provisions included in the ACA that were not part of the EJA or NH Transparency and Improvement Act fit within the overall goal of strengthening facility accountability and quality improvement. One provision calls for a value-based purchasing program for skilled nursing facilities, the development of indicators of quality and efficiency in these demonstration facilities, and making measures available to the public. CMS is already implementing this demonstration for Medicare payments to skilled nursing facilities, with the expectation that improvements in quality may reduce hospitalizations and create a savings pool. The four performance domains that CMS developed are staffing, hospitalization, select outcomes based on Minimum Data Set assessment data, and survey deficiencies. NHs with an overall quality score in the top 20% and the top 20% in terms of improvement in their scores will be eligible for a share of the savings pool. Another provision modifies the skilled nursing facilities prospective payment system to allow for changes in the "look back period" to ensure that only services provided to a resident after admission are used in the resident case mix classification that determines a facility's Medicare payment rate.

Other Facility Staff Provisions

There were several provisions in the ACA related to NH staff, in addition to the reporting requirements included in the transparency mandates. The ACA specifies that the nurse aide certification training must include information on dementia and management of the consequences, as well as training to identify and prevent resident abuse. It also requires national criminal background checks for staff involved in direct resident care, provides an appeal process for employees who are dismissed or not hired as a result of background checks, and prohibits hiring of abusive workers. Two EJA provisions in the ACA call for creating a national registry for certified nursing assistants that would list individuals barred from NH employment because of a history of abuse of older persons and grants and other incentives for individuals to seek employment and training in LTC.

Enforcement and Quality Assurance Mechanisms

There were several enforcement provisions in the ACA addressing improvements to the complaint process, the use of CMPs, a pilot program to monitor the performance of large chains, and a series of EJA initiatives aimed at strengthening state and federal initiatives to prevent, detect, and resolve elder abuse in NHs. The ACA requires that states enact a complaint resolution process that will track all complaints, determine their severity, and specify investigative protocols as well as establish and adhere to timelines for responding. It also authorizes creation of a standardized form for use by complainants, although oral complaints will be allowed, and complaints may be filed either with the state survey or ombudsman programs.

The increased fines proposed by Senators Grassley and Kohl in S. 2461 were stripped out of the 2009 bill; however, the remaining provisions on CMPs allows for a reduction of CMPs if a facility self-reports and promptly corrects the deficiency, unless it is a repeat citation or reflects a pattern of harm, widespread harm, immediate jeopardy, or a resident's death. In addition, informal dispute resolution processes will be allowed even after penalties are imposed, but the fine may be placed in an escrow account until the dispute is resolved. Finally, CMP funds collected from facilities would be used for quality improvement benefiting residents, broadly defined. The legislation authorizes a demonstration project "to develop, test, and implement an independent monitor program to oversee interstate and large intrastate chains" of NHs as well. The focus would be on chains with "serious safety and quality of care problems."

Two additional EJA provisions allocate funding for grants and training focusing on abuse and neglect for ombudsmen and staff of adult protective services agencies, provide grants to improve state survey agencies' complaint investigation systems, and establish a national training institute for federal and state surveyors to improve surveyor training in abuse and neglect. As noted above, a provision also authorizes the creation of a national nurse aide registry.

IMPLEMENTATION

For decades, NH reform occurred only on the heels of a scandal, one sufficiently dramatic to attract public attention and generate a demand for reform.

This, for example, is how the original requirement for sprinklers in NHs arose—the result of horrific multiple fire deaths. However, the major NH reforms in the ACA and those in OBRA '87 took a different path. They followed what might be called the "hitchhiker model." Both of these major reform packages were attached to another stronger legislative cause. While this attachment to a larger, stronger bill worked in securing passage for the EJA, NH Transparency and Improvement Act, and other NH provisions, their political vulnerability remains as implementation begins to unfold.

Even before incorporation into the ACA, the most contentious part of the NH Transparency and Improvement Act—the increase in the size and certainty of large fines for seriously substandard care—was defeated by the NH industry and removed from the 2008 bill. While CMS has made significant progress implementing the remaining provisions in a timely fashion, the industry has still sought to "chip away" at the provisions, seeking to weaken them in the implementation phase. Take the requirement to make public the result of complaint investigations, for example, including those about abuse. Here, the industry has sought to weaken the public reporting of deficiencies and penalties in a variety of ways, such as limiting public notice of substantiated complaints about abuse (e.g., excluding facility reports of "incidents" of abuse). Similarly, at the same time the ACA reforms were being adopted, the AHCA was quietly circulating a proposal on Capitol Hill to repeal the statutory requirement for annual surveys of nursing facilities and to go back to the Reagan Administration's 1982 proposal for less-than-annual surveys. Strengthening the survey process and enforcement have always been contentious issues, and the AHCA and AQNHC have a history of successfully delaying implementation or substantially weakening such efforts even when advocates have succeeded in the legislative arena (Edelman, 1997–1998). Thus, consumer advocates recognize that the legislative victory against a powerful and well-funded industry group is one stage of a continuing struggle, even with the ACA.

For the components of the ACA associated with the EJA, the lack of sufficient urgency to ensure its passage between 2002 and 2009 plays out now in several ways. For example, the Administration on Aging has not yet meaningfully established the Elder Justice Coordinating Council or appointed people to the Council's Advisory Committee, although this was a key element in the bill and was intended to oversee implementation of the EJA's broader provisions. Similarly, advocates have not been able to get adequate funding from Congress to implement the EJA. Indeed, "the major challenge," according to Lindberg et al. (2011, p. 115), "will be advocating to ensure that Congress actually appropriates the monies authorized." The passage of the ACA was only a cease-fire with respect to health reform in general (Miller, 2010), and so it is for the EJA and NH Transparency and Improvement Act provisions. The fundamental battles will remain, albeit with some important gains for advocates.

REFERENCES

Acierno, R., Hernandez, M. A., Amstadter, A. B., Resnick, H. S., Steve, K., Muzzy, W., & Kilpatrick, D. G. (2010). Prevalence and correlates of emotional, physical, sexual, and financial abuse and potential neglect in the United States: The National Elder Mistreatment Study. *American Journal of Public Health, 100*(2), 292–297.

Bonnie, R. J., & Wallace, R. B. (Eds.). (2002). *Elder mistreatment: Abuse, neglect, and exploitation in an aging America. Panel to Review Risk and Prevalence of Elder Abuse and Neglect, National Research Council*. Washington, DC: National Academies Press.

Center for Medicare Advocacy. (2010). *Health reform: The nursing home provisions.* CMA Alert. June 17. Retrieved from http://www.medicareadvocacy.org/2010/06/17/health-reform-provisions/

Duhigg, C. (2007). At many homes, more profit and less nursing. *New York Times.* September 23. Retrieved from http://www.nytimes.com/2007/09/23/business/23nursing.html?_r=2&oref=slogin

Edelman, T. (1997–1998). The politics of long-term care at the federal level and implications for quality. *Generations, 21*(4), 37–41.

Gagel, B. (1995). Health care quality improvement project. *Health Care Financing Review, 16*(4), 15–23.

Harrington, C., Olney, B., Carrillo, H., & Kang, T. (2011). Nurse staffing and deficiencies in the largest for-profit nursing home chains and chains owned by private equity companies. *Health Services Research.* doi: 10.1111/j.1475-6773.2011.01311.x

Hawes, C., Phillips, C. D., Morris, J. N., Mor, V., Fries, B., Steele–Freidlob, E., . . . Nennsteil, M. (1997). The impact of OBRA-87 and the RAI on indicators of process quality in nursing homes. *Journal of the American Geriatrics Society, 45*(8), 977–985.

Kumar, V., Norton, E. C., & Encinosa, W. E. (2006). OBRA 1987 and the quality of nursing home care. *International Journal of Health Care Finance and Economics, 6*(1), 49–81.

Lindberg, B. W., Sabatino, C. P., & Blancato, R. B. (2011). Bringing national action to a national disgrace: The history of the Elder Justice Act. *National Academy of Elder Law Attorneys Journal, 7*(1), 105–124.

Miller, T. P. (2010). Health reform: Only a cease-fire. *Health Affairs, 29*(6), 1101–1105.

Mixson, P. M. (2010). Public policy, elder abuse, and adult protective services: The struggle for coherence. *Journal of Elder Abuse and Neglect, 22*(1–2), 16–36.

Mor, V., Intrator, O., Hiris, J., Fries, B., Phillips, C. D., Hawes, C.,. . . Morris, J. N. (1997). Impact of the MDS on changes in nursing home discharge rates and destinations. *Journal of the American Geriatrics Society, 45*(8), 1002–1010.

Oberlander, J. (2010). Long time coming: Why health reform finally passed. *Health Affairs, 29*(6), 1112–1116. doi: 10.1377/hlthaff.2010.0447

Pear, R. (2008). Serious deficiencies in nursing homes are often missed, report says. *New York Times*, 23, May 15.

Phillips, C. D., Morris, J. N., Hawes, C., Mor, V., Fries, B., Murphy, K., . . . Nennsteil, M.. (1997). The impact of the RAI on ADLs, continence, communication, cognition, and psychosocial well-being. *Journal of the American Geriatrics Society*, *45*(8), 986–993.

Reichard, J. B. (2008, May 15). Worries over nursing home care agitate law-makers. CQ HealthBeat. Retrieved from http://www.commonwealthfund.org/Newsletters/Washington-Health-Policy-in-Review/2008/May/Washington-Health-Policy-Week-in-Review---May-2008/Worries-Over-Nursing-Home-Care-Agitate-Lawmakers.aspx

Schulte, B. (2008). A bill aims for nursing home reform: Proposed legislation con-siders the biggest reform of the industry in decades. *U.S. News & World Report*. February 22. Retrieved fromwww.usnews.com/news/national/articles/2008/02/22/a-bill-aims-for-nursing-home-reform

Singer, P. (2008). Members offered many bills but passed few. *Roll Call*. December 1. Retrieved from http://www.rollcall.com/issues/54_61/30466-1.html

Teaster, P. B., Wangmo, T., & Anetzberger, G. J. (2010). A glass half full: The dubious history of elder abuse policy. *Journal of Elder Abuse and Neglect*, *22*(1–2), 6–15. doi: 10.1080/08946560903436130

United States House Select Committee on Aging, Subcommittee on Health and Long-Term Care. (1985). *Elder abuse: A national disgrace*. 99th Congress, 1st session, 99–502.Washington, DC: Government Printing Office.

United States House Select Committee on Aging, Subcommittee on Health and Long-Term Care. (1990). *Elder abuse: A decade of shame and inaction*.101st Congress, 2nd session. Washington, DC: Government Printing Office.

United States House Select Committee on Aging, Subcommittee on Health and Long-Term Care. (1991). *Protecting America's abused elderly: The need for Congressional action*.102nd Congress, 1st session. Washington, DC: Government Printing Office.

United States House Committee on Government Reform, Special Investigations Division. (2001). *Abuse of residents is a major problem in U.S. nursing homes*. H. A. Waxman. 107th Congress, 1st session. Washington, DC: Government Printing Office.

United States Senate Special Committee on Aging. (2009). *Senators reintroduce bill to raise standard of care in nursing homes nationwide* [press release]. March 19. Retrieved from http://aging.senate.gov/hearing_detail.cfm?id=310113&

United States Senate Special Committee on Aging. (2011, March 2). *Justice for all: Ending elder abuse, neglect and financial exploitation*. Retrieved from http://aging.senate.gov/hearing_detail.cmf?id=33155&

United States Department of Health and Human Services, Office of Inspector General. (2006). *Nursing home complaint investigations*. OEI-01-04-00340, July 2006.

United States Government Accountability Office. (1999). *Nursing homes: Additional steps needed to strengthen enforcement of federal quality standards* (GAO/HEHS-99-46). Washington, DC: U.S. Government Printing Office.

United States Government Accountability Office. (2003). *Nursing home qual-ity: Prevalence of serious problems, while declining, reinforces importance of enhanced oversight*. GAO-03-561. Washington, DC: U.S. Government Printing Office. July 15.

United States Government Accountability Office. (2005). *Nursing homes: Despite increased oversight, challenges remain in ensuring high-quality care and resident safety.* GAO-06-117. Washington, DC: U.S. Government Printing Office. December 28.

United States Government Accountability Office. (2007). *Nursing home reform: Continued attention is needed to improve quality of care in small but significant share of homes.*GAO-07-794T. Washington, DC: U.S. Government Printing Office. May 2.

United States Government Accountability Office. (2008). *Nursing homes: Federal monitoring surveys demonstrate continued understatement of serious care problems and CMS oversight weaknesses.* GAO-08-517. Washington, DC: U.S. Government Printing Office. May 9.

United States Government Accountability Office. (2009). *Medicare and Medicaid participating facilities: CMS needs to reexamine its approach for funding state oversight of health care facilities.* GAO-09-64. Washington, DC: U.S. Government Printing Office. February 13.

United States Government Accountability Office. (2011). *Stronger federal leadership could help improve response to elder abuse.*Washington, DC: U.S. Government Printing Office. GAO-11-384T, Mar 2.

Care Coordination for Dually Eligible Medicare-Medicaid Beneficiaries Under the Affordable Care Act

DAVID C. GRABOWSKI, PhD

Associate Professor, Department of Health Policy, Harvard Medical School, Boston, Massachusetts, USA

The coordination of Medicare and Medicaid benefits and services for dually eligible enrollees has been a longstanding policy challenge. Several provisions of the Affordable Care Act (ACA) attempt to address this lack of coordination, including the establishment of the Federal Coordinated Health Care Office. This paper reviews the major changes under the ACA directed at care coordination for the dually eligible population and then concludes with a discussion of the continuing legislative and legal challenges in integrating care for the dually eligible.

OVERVIEW OF THE POLICY PROBLEM

Individuals who are dually eligible for both Medicare and Medicaid have received considerable policy attention in recent years due to their high cost and complex health needs. Research suggests that the dually eligible comprise the sickest, poorest, and most costly cohort of beneficiaries in the nation's health care system (Bruen & Holahan, 2003; Reese, 2009). Although this population is relatively small in number, consisting of approximately 9 million individuals, spending on dually eligible accounts for roughly 36% of Medicare's total spending and 39% of Medicaid's spending (Kaiser Family

Foundation, 2011a). Mainly because of their poor health status and continual health care needs, the Medicare costs of dually eligible beneficiaries are 1.5 times those of other Medicare beneficiaries (Medicare Payment Advisory Commission, 2004).

The poor coordination of Medicare and Medicaid benefits and services has been a long-standing problem in the care of the dual-eligible population (Ryan & Super, 2003). The fragmented coverage of these services often contributes to higher costs and worse patient outcomes. In a recent presentation, the Centers for Medicare and Medicaid Services (CMS; 2011) contrasted nonintegrated and integrated care models for dually eligible individuals. Without integrated care, enrollees have three ID cards (Medicare, prescription drugs, Medicaid), three different sets of benefits, and multiple providers who rarely communicate. As such, care is not well-coordinated, and enrollees are likely candidates for further health decline and nursing home placement. With integrated care, enrollees have one ID card with a single set of comprehensive benefits covering primary, acute, prescription drug, and long-term care. They have an individualized care plan with a coordinated team of health providers. Ideally, this integrated care can be delivered in a community setting, which is consistent with the majority of enrollees' preferences.

An important example of a poor outcome under our current, poorly coordinated system of care is the inappropriate hospitalization of dually eligible individuals (Grabowski, Stewart, Broderick, & Coots, 2008). Medicaid is the dominant payer of long-term care services for the dually eligible, while Medicare is the primary payer for hospital services. Thus, Medicaid programs do not typically provide long-term care providers with an incentive to eliminate inappropriate hospitalizations. Walsh et al. (2010) found that of the 1.6 million persons who were dually eligible for Medicaid and Medicare in 2005, more than one-third of them in long-term care or skilled nursing facility settings were hospitalized from these settings at least once, totaling almost 1 million hospitalizations. Of these hospitalizations, 39% were deemed avoidable, either because the condition precipitating it could have been prevented or because the condition could have been treated in a lower level of care. Ultimately, the authors estimated that the Medicare program spent $3 billion in 2005 on potentially avoidable hospitalizations for dually eligible beneficiaries, while the Medicaid program spent $463 million on these hospitalizations.

CONCEPTUAL FRAMEWORK: THE ROLE OF FINANCING AND PAYMENT IN CARE COORDINATION

The coordination of health care services at the delivery level relates directly to the financing and payment of those services (Leutz, 1999). At the financing level, the presence of multiple payers in health care is known to introduce conflicting incentives for providers, which may have negative implications for cost containment, service delivery, and quality of care (Grabowski, 2007; Ng, Harrington, & Kitchener, 2010). The fundamental issue is that the actions of one payer may affect the costs and outcomes of patients covered by other payers. These "external" costs and benefits can occur both within and across health care settings, and little incentive exists for a payer to incorporate these externalities into payment and coverage decisions. As a result, the behaviors of health care payers—even public payers—often deviate substantially from the social optimum. For example, under the traditional benefit structure for dually eligible persons, little incentive exists for state Medicaid programs to enact policies to lower Medicare-financed hospitalizations because they do not accrue any of the potential savings (Grabowski, O'Malley, & Barhydt, 2007). Indeed, state Medicaid programs often enact policies such as bed-hold payments that increase hospital and post-acute expenditures for the Medicare program (Intrator et al., 2007). A model that blends Medicare and Medicaid financing introduces a stronger incentive to minimize transitions for dually eligible beneficiaries from Medicaid-financed nursing home care, for example, to higher-cost Medicare-financed hospital care.

Payment structure also has implications for the coordination of care. Cost shifting occurs for reasons beyond the fragmentation of financing across programs. For example, the high rate of 30-day hospital readmissions from Medicare-financed skilled nursing facilities is an example of poor coordination *within* the Medicare program (Mor, Intrator, Feng, & Grabowski, 2010). Traditional fee-for-service payment creates little incentive for providers to manage the volume and intensity of services, because providers are rewarded with greater revenue when they deliver more services. In the case of 30-day readmissions, hospitals are rewarded with higher revenue when beneficiaries bounce back to the hospital. Through risk-based capitation, managed care potentially encourages more efficient care delivery (Miller & Weissert, 2004; Tritz, 2006; Tumlinson, Reester, & Missmar, 2003; Walsh & Clark, 2002). Under this model, a single entity receives a fixed predetermined monthly payment (i.e., capitation rate), which provides the incentive to minimize wasteful care. Ideally, under capitation, hospitals would not be rewarded when individuals are readmitted. Similarly, other risk-based models such as accountable care organizations (ACOs), bundled payment, global budgeting, and medical homes also provide similar incentives to coordinate care in ways that could reduce inefficient service use.

With respect to care delivery, the coordination of financing and payment can be thought of as necessary, but not sufficient, conditions for the coordination of services. For example, at the delivery level, care coordination activities might include case management, team-based care models, patient education, management of care transitions, communication protocols for providers, and shared clinical and social information. However, without an alignment in payment and financing in which providers can internalize the costs and benefits of their actions, we have little reason to suspect any sustainable coordination in service delivery at the ground level.

Prior Evidence and Experience With Care Coordination

Care coordination is often justified as a "win-win," with the idea that it will improve both quality and access while also lowering costs. The evidence to date on care coordination suggests this goal is not easily achievable. The CMS Medicare Care Coordination Demonstration, a randomized evaluation of 15 care coordination programs including 18,309 fee-for-service enrollees, concluded that care coordination holds little promise of reducing expenditures for chronically ill beneficiaries (Peikes, Chen, Schore, & Brown, 2009). Similarly, managed care programs that blend Medicare and Medicaid financing have also shown mixed results (Grabowski, 2006).

The Program of All-Inclusive Care for the Elderly (PACE) and Minnesota Senior Health Options (MSHO) programs are the only two models integrating Medicaid and Medicare that have been rigorously evaluated. The evaluations of PACE (White, Abel, & Kidder, 2000) and MSHO (Kane & Homyak, 2003) both found higher program costs relative to comparison groups. Factors potentially underlying this result include the failure to target services effectively to enrollees via a stringent preadmission process and the inability to contain spending on particular services. Quality of care and enrollees' access to services were found to improve under PACE (Chatterji, Burstein, Kidder, & White, 1998) and remain relatively stable under MSHO (Kane et al., 2005; Kane, Homyak, Bershadsky, Lum, & Siadaty, 2003). Although PACE was designated as a permanent Medicare program in 1997, growth in the number of PACE programs and enrollment has been relatively slow (Gross, Temkin-Greener, Kunitz, & Mukamel, 2004).

Thus, the results to date suggest that if we want better quality for the sickest and most vulnerable patients, it may cost more. The key question from an economic standpoint is whether we are getting "value" from additional expenditures in terms of increased access to services, quality of care, and quality of life. From a policy perspective, we often work under the "budget neutrality" restriction in which any additional programs expenditures must be offset by program savings. Based on the evidence to date, coordinated care programs, especially those with voluntary enrollment, may not be able to generate cost offsets. That said, these programs have great promise toward improving access and quality for dually eligible beneficiaries.

One recent policy directed at the dually eligible was the authorization of Medicare Advantage special needs plans (SNPs) under the Medicare Modernization Act of 2003, with the idea of attracting a different type of beneficiary into Medicare Advantage (Grabowski, 2009). From the perspective of program coordination, SNPs allow states the opportunity to combine Medicare and Medicaid managed care contracting for dually eligible beneficiaries without having to secure special Medicare demonstration authority from CMS. However, SNP enrollment has been relatively modest to date, likely reflecting the fact that—unless SNPs contract with state Medicaid programs to offer a coordinated product—these plans may offer little additional value to dually eligible beneficiaries relative to traditional Medicare Advantage plans (Bishop, Leutz, Gurewich, Ryan, & Thomas, 2007; Verdier, Gold, & Davis, 2008).

The Medicare Improvements for Patients and Providers Act (MIPPA) of 2008 required new dually eligible SNPs—starting in 2010—to have contracts with state Medicaid agencies. Existing dually eligible SNPs that did not have a contract with the state were allowed to continue to operate but could not expand into new service areas. Following MIPPA, much of the onus now falls to state Medicaid programs to engage SNPs in new partnerships to increase the number of dually eligible beneficiaries enrolled in joint Medicare-Medicaid products.

Moving forward, the evidence on Medicare-Medicaid integration would greatly benefit from more sophisticated analyses that appropriately address the issue of selection into a program. That is, individuals enrolling in integrated programs (i.e., the treatment group) may be different in ways unobservable to the researcher compared with individuals not enrolling in these programs (i.e., the control group). These unobservable differences may ultimately bias comparisons of costs and health outcomes across the two study groups. Clearly, the gold standard here would be a randomized study design. When randomization is viewed as too costly or infeasible, an instrumental variables approach can also be used to address the issue of selection. By finding an instrument that predicts program enrollment but not the outcomes of interest such as costs and health outcomes, this approach can be used effectively to "randomize" individuals even in a voluntary program.

Changes included in the Affordable Care Act (ACA) HR 4972 (Public Law 111–148 and 111–152) will attempt to improve the coordination of services for dually eligible individuals (Thorpe & Philyaw, 2010). Moreover, they have the opportunity to increase the quality of the evidence base around these programs. This paper first summarizes the key changes under the legislation before offering some recommendations for policymakers in terms of next steps following the ACA.

CARE COORDINATION FOR THE DUALLY ELIGIBLE UNDER HEALTH CARE REFORM

To address the growing needs of the dually eligible and to stem rising health care costs, the ACA (Section 2602) mandated that the secretary of the Department of Health and Human Services establish a Federal Coordinated Health Care Office (FCHCO) within CMS. The purpose of the FCHCO (or the

"Duals Office") is to increase quality, decrease costs, and improve access and care coordination for dually eligible individuals by integrating various services in order to eliminate redundancy and friction between Medicare and Medicaid.

The major areas of focus for the FCHCO include program alignment, data and analytics, and models and demonstrations. Program alignment includes any issues that arise from the lack of cohesiveness between Medicare and Medicaid. The data and analytics objective will focus on leveraging, standardizing, and sharing data so that both the federal and state governments can improve coordination of services. The models and demonstrations objective will consist of research, design, and implementation of dual eligibility–related demonstrations and the management of analytics. In addition to researching and testing new models of care, the office will also seek to promote the use of existing models that have proved successful and eliminate those models that have been unsuccessful in order to improve the functioning of payment and delivery systems. This objective will be undertaken in conjunction with the Center for Medicare and Medicaid Innovation (CMMI) (established under Section 3021 of the ACA). The CMMI will evaluate the effectiveness of various payment and care models in order to improve the delivery of quality care to dually eligible individuals and also to reduce costs related to care for the dually eligible population.

CMS is currently undertaking several demonstrations that are being developed by the FCHCO and the CMMI in order to facilitate care integration for dually eligible beneficiaries. The State Demonstration to Integrate Care for Dual Eligible Individuals has awarded 15 states $1 million each to implement person-centered care models that fully coordinate primary, acute, behavioral health, and long-term care services for dually eligible individuals. The following states have been selected to develop their demonstration proposals: California, Colorado, Connecticut, Massachusetts, Michigan, Minnesota, New York, North Carolina, Oklahoma, Oregon, South Carolina, Tennessee, Vermont, Washington, and Wisconsin.

The demonstration proposals offer 15 different state-based "laboratories" among which comparisons may be made to evaluate differences in program spending and health outcomes. Although the demonstration proposals are subject to change during the demonstration design and implementation process, the proposals submitted to CMS include variations in service delivery models, target populations, benefits packages, financing, beneficiary protections, and stakeholder involvement (Kaiser Family Foundation, 2011b). Thus, these 15 state demonstrations have significant potential to provide new evidence on the cost-effectiveness of integrated care models.

The Independence at Home demonstration was mandated by Section 3024 of the ACA to test a payment incentive and service delivery model that utilizes physician- and nurse practitioner–directed home-based primary care teams with the goal of reducing expenditures and improving health outcomes. This 3-year demonstration, which was scheduled to begin on January 1, 2012, will target high-cost patients with two or more chronic illnesses, a non-elective hospital admission over the past 12 months, acute or subacute rehabilitation services over the past 12 months, and two or more functional dependencies requiring the assistance of another person. The incentive payments are subject to performance by the medical groups on a series of quality measures, including a measure of care coordination. A practice will be eligible to receive a payment if actual expenditures for a year for the applicable beneficiaries enrolled are less than the estimated spending target.

The ACA legislation also contained a number of other new delivery models that might lead to improved coordination of services among the dually eligible including health homes for the chronically ill (Section 2703), integration of hospital and physician care (Section 2704), value-based payment modifier for physicians (Section 3007), accountable care organizations (Section 3022), bundled payment demonstration (Section 3023), hospital readmissions reduction program (Section 3025), support for medical homes (Section 3502), and medication management (Section 3503). Finally, Section 3205 in the ACA legislation extended the authority of SNPs through December 31, 2013.

CARE COORDINATION BEYOND HEALTH CARE REFORM

Many of the initiatives for coordinating care under the ACA legislation are still quite nascent and unformed. The evaluations of the integrated care demonstrations and the Independence at Home demonstrations will provide important new evidence on care coordination models. This section highlights four principles that will factor into the success of these and future coordinated care initiatives: the pairing of delivery and payment reforms, the engagement of Medicaid, blending of Medicare-Medicaid financing, and enrollment in managed care.

Pairing Delivery and Payment Reforms

A large number of the reforms under the ACA target either care delivery (e.g., medical homes, medication management) or payment (e.g., bundling, value-based purchasing) but not both. In the delivery-only models, the underlying financial incentives are not changed, which may impact program sustainability in the longer-term. For example, it is unclear whether providers implementing medical homes or medication management would sustain these initiatives after the conclusion of the CMS demonstration because these delivery-only models often do not compel providers to internalize the costs and benefits of their actions. In the payment-only models, the financial incentives may be correctly aligned, but at the delivery level, care may not be meaningfully coordinated. For instance, the evidence to date suggests that even when SNPs have blended Medicare-Medicaid financing, they often do not have coordinated services. Similar concerns may exist with bundled payment and value-based purchasing models. The Independence at Home demonstration is obviously an important exception in that it pairs both delivery and payment reforms.

Engaging Medicaid

Several of the policy reforms in the ACA that have received considerable attention are largely Medicare-only solutions that fail to engage Medicaid. For example, bundling and ACOs are two such ACA reforms. The ACO model establishes local delivery collaborations (e.g., primary care practices, specialty groups, hospitals, skilled nursing facilities) that can generate shared savings relative to a Medicare spending benchmark based on expected expenditures (Fisher et al., 2009). Bundling introduces global Medicare payments shared across multiple providers to incentivize more efficient resource use. Under these systems, a hospital and skilled nursing facility, for example, might share in the savings from preventing a Medicare hospital readmission. As such, a hospital would have less incentive to discharge a patient prematurely to a skilled nursing facility and the skilled nursing facility would have less incentive to rehospitalize the patient.

Although bundling and ACOs have promise toward targeting inefficient health care expenditures, a major issue with the dually eligible population is the failure to target or otherwise include Medicaid long-term care expenditures. Some of the current inefficiencies in Medicare spending for the dually eligible population relate to state Medicaid policies. For example, Grabowski, Feng, Intrator, and Mor (2010) found that variation in Medicare skilled nursing facility rehospitalizations was related to the generosity of Medicaid nursing home bed-hold policies. Because a Medicare-only solution such as ACOs and bundling will not take into account of potential spillovers from Medicaid, reforms will have a lower probability of success without engagement from the states (Grabowski, 2007).

Blending of Medicare and Medicaid Financing

One dramatic proposal to address the conflicting financial incentives across Medicare and Medicaid is to shift financial responsibility for the care of the dually eligible population to the federal government or to the states (Holahan & Weil, 2007; U.S. General Accounting Office, 1995). The idea of federalizing (or defederalizing) care for dually eligible enrollees dates back at least to the early 1980s (U.S. General Accounting Office, 1995). The idea is that this shift—either to Medicare or Medicaid—would eliminate the misaligned financial incentives for dually eligible enrollees. Importantly, the shifting of responsibilities from Medicaid to Medicare (or Medicaid to Medicare) would address the conflicting financial incentives across the two programs but would not (necessarily) address the lack of care coordination or other problems currently present in the system.

Although either program could—in theory—take financial responsibility for the duals, Medicare is a national program administered by the federal government, with broader taxing and borrowing authority. State revenues can often be quite volatile. Given the cross-state variation in Medicaid eligibility and benefits, defederalization also raises important concerns in terms of equity across states.

Even without full federalization (or defederalization), other options are present to blend Medicare and Medicaid financing such as a shared savings approach (Rosenbaum, Thorpe, & Schroth, 2009). Under the ACA, shared savings models between the state and the federal government were proposed in several of the integrated care demonstration proposals (e.g., Connecticut). Other demonstration states (e.g., Michigan) proposed to take on the full Medicare financial risk by receiving a risk-adjusted Medicare capitation from CMS and unifying Medicare and Medicaid at the state level.

Compulsory Enrollment in Managed Care

The President's Deficit Commission recently recommended placing all dually eligible persons in a combined Medicaid–managed care product (National Commission on Fiscal Responsibility and Reform, 2010). Presumably, this approach would both change the financial and delivery incentives present in the system. This proposed approach would give Medicaid full responsibility for providing health coverage for the dually eligible. The rationale for running the program through Medicaid is that it has a larger system of managed care than Medicare, which would theoretically result in better care coordination and administrative simplicity. Medicare would still continue to pay its share of costs by reimbursing Medicaid. The commission estimated that this reform would save $1 billion in 2015 and $12 billion through 2020.

A mandatory Medicaid–managed care system in Arizona was found to generate potential Medicaid savings for long-term care beneficiaries relative to a Medicaid fee-for-service system (McCall & Korb, 1997; Weissert, Lesnick, Musliner, & Foley, 1997). Although this approach has potential, a model that also included mandatory Medicare enrollment would likely be challenged on both legal and political grounds. Medicare's freedom of choice provision provides beneficiaries with the statutory right to choose between a managed Medicare program and Medicare fee-for-service. Politically, advocates have raised concerns that managed care will mean that the dually eligible will have to change doctors, go to new locations for care, and have fewer choices (Peters, 2005).

CONCLUSION

In sum, the current structure of Medicare and Medicaid does not offer a coordinated system of care for the majority of dually eligible beneficiaries, creating a number of conflicting incentives across the two programs. These conflicting incentives often lead to increased program costs for Medicare and Medicaid, a lack of care management, and poor quality of care. The ACA contains a number of important provisions toward improving the coordination of benefits and services for dually eligible enrollees, including the establishment of a new office within CMS, the introduction of demonstrations to pilot new delivery and payment models, and the extension of the Medicare Advantage SNPs.

Although these developments are encouraging, policy makers will face a number of further legislative and legal challenges in integrating care for the dually eligible. These challenges include the pairing of payment and delivery reforms, the need to engage Medicaid, the feasibility of federalizing Medicaid (or defederalizing Medicare), and compulsory enrollment in managed care. With the aging baby boom generation and projected budget shortfalls at the federal and state levels, the care of the dually eligible population will be a continued area of interest to policymakers in the coming decades.

REFERENCES

Bishop, C., Leutz, W., Gurewich, D., Ryan, M., & Thomas, C. (2007). *Medicare special care needs plans: Lessons from dual-eligible demonstrations for CMS, states, health plans, and providers.* Waltham. MA: Brandeis University.

Bruen, B., & Holahan, J. (2003). *Shifting the cost of dual eligibles: Implications for states and the federal government.* Menlo Park, CA: The Henry J. Kaiser Family Foundation.

Centers for Medicaid and Medicare Services. (2011). *Integrating care for dual eligibles.* Retrieved from www.cms.gov/DualEligible/Downloads/DualsOfficePresentation2011.pdf

Chatterji, P., Burstein, N. R., Kidder, D., & White, A. (1998). *Evaluation of the Program of All-Inclusive Care for the Elderly (PACE) demonstration: The impact of PACE on participant outcomes* (No. HCFA Contract #500-96-0003/TO4). Cambridge, MA: Abt Associates Inc.

Fisher, E. S., McClellan, M. B., Bertko, J., Lieberman, S. M., Lee, J. J., Lewis, J. L., & Skinner, J. S. (2009). Fostering accountable health care: Moving forward in Medicare. *Health Affairs (Millwood), 28*(2), w219–w231.

Grabowski, D. C. (2006). The cost-effectiveness of noninstitutional long-term care services: Review and synthesis of the most recent evidence. *Medical Care Research and Review, 63*(1), 3–28.

Grabowski, D. C. (2007). Medicare and Medicaid: Conflicting incentives for long-term care. *Milbank Quarterly, 85*(4), 579–610.

Grabowski, D. C. (2009). Special needs plans and the coordination of benefits and services for dual eligibles. *Health Affairs (Millwood)*, *28*(1), 136–146.

Grabowski, D. C., Feng, Z., Intrator, O., & Mor, V. (2010). Medicaid bed-hold policy and Medicare skilled nursing facility rehospitalizations. *Health Services Research*, *45*(6 Pt 2), 1963–1980.

Grabowski, D. C., O'Malley, A. J., & Barhydt, N. R. (2007). The costs and potential savings associated with nursing home hospitalizations. *Health Affairs*, *26*(6), 1753–1761.

Grabowski, D. C., Stewart, K. A., Broderick, S. M., & Coots, L. A. (2008). Predictors of nursing home hospitalization: A review of the literature. *Medical Care Research and Review*, *65*(1), 3–39.

Gross, D. L., Temkin-Greener, H., Kunitz, S., & Mukamel, D. B. (2004). The growing pains of integrated health care for the elderly: Lessons from the expansion of PACE. *Milbank Quarterly*, *82*(2), 257–282.

Holahan, J., & Weil, A. (2007). Toward real Medicaid reform. *Health Affairs (Millwood)*, *26*(2), w254–w270.

Intrator, O., Grabowski, D. C., Zinn, J., Schleinitz, M., Feng, Z., Miller, S., & Mor, V. (2007). Hospitalization of nursing home residents: The effects of states' Medicaid payment and bed-hold policies. *Health Services Research*, *42*(4), 1651–1671.

Kaiser Family Foundation. (2011a). *The role of Medicare for the people dually eligible for Medicare and Medicaid* (No. 8138). Washington, DC: Author.

Kaiser Family Foundation. (2011b). *Proposed models to integrate Medicare and Medicaid benefits for dual eligibles: A look at the 15 state design contracts funded by CMS*. Washington, DC: Author.

Kane, R. L., & Homyak, P. (2003). *Multistate Evaluation of Dual Eligibles demonstration: Minnesota Senior Health Options Evaluation Focusing on Utilization, Cost, and Quality of Care: Final Report* (HCFA Contract No. 500-96-0008). Baltimore, MD: Centers for Medicare and Medicaid Services.

Kane, R. L., Homyak, P., Bershadsky, B., Lum, T., Flood, S., & Zhang, H. (2005). The quality of care under a managed-care program for dual eligibles. *Gerontologist*, *45*(4), 496–504.

Kane, R. L., Homyak, P., Bershadsky, B., Lum, Y. S., & Siadaty, M. S. (2003). Outcomes of managed care of dually eligible older persons. *Gerontologist*, *43*(2), 165–174.

Leutz, W. N. (1999). Five laws for integrating medical and social services: Lessons from the United States and the United Kingdom. *Milbank Quarterly*, *77*(1), 77–110, iv–v.

McCall, N., & Korb, J. (1997). Utilization of services in Arizona's capitated Medicaid program for long-term care beneficiaries. *Health Care Financing Review*, *19*(2), 119–134. Medicare Payment Advisory Commission. (2004). *Report to the Congress: Medicare payment policy*. Washington, DC: Medicare Payment Advisory Commission.

Miller, E., & Weissert, W. G. (2004). Managed care for Medicare-Medicaid dual eligibles: Appropriateness, availability, payment, and policy. *Journal of Applied Gerontology*, *23*(4), 333–348.

Mor, V., Intrator, O., Feng, Z., & Grabowski, D. C. (2010). The revolving door of rehospitalization from skilled nursing facilities. *Health Affairs (Millwood)*, *29*(1), 57–64.

National Commission on Fiscal Responsibility and Reform. (2010). *The moment of truth: Report of the National Commission on Fiscal Responsibility and Reform.* Washington, DC: Author.

Ng, T., Harrington, C., & Kitchener, M. (2010). Medicare and Medicaid in long-term care. *Health Affairs (Millwood), 29*(1), 22–28.

Peikes, D., Chen, A., Schore, J., & Brown, R. (2009). Effects of care coordination on hospitalization, quality of care, and health care expenditures among Medicare beneficiaries: 15 randomized trials. *Journal of the American Medical Association, 301*(6), 603–618.

Peters, C. P. (2005). *Medicare Advantage SNPs: A new opportunity for integrated care?* (No. Issue Brief #808). Washington, DC: National Health Policy Forum.

Reese, S. (2009). Dual eligibles best served with coordinated benefit design. *Managed Healthcare Executive, 19*(1), 25–26.

Rosenbaum, S., Thorpe, J. H., & Schroth, S. (2009). *Supporting alternative integrated models for dual eligibles: A legal analysis of current and future option.* Policy Brief. Hamilton, NJ: Center for Health Care Strategies, Inc.

Ryan, J., & Super, N. (2003). *Dually eligible for Medicare and Medicaid: Two for one or double jeopardy?* Washington, DC: National Health Policy Forum.

Thorpe, K. E., & Philyaw, M. (2010). Impact of health care reform on Medicare and dual Medicare-Medicaid beneficiaries. *The Cancer Journal, 16*(6), 584–587 doi:510.1097/PPO.1090b1013e3181ff3156

Tritz, K. (2006). *Integrating Medicare and Medicaid services through managed care.* Washington, DC: Congressional Research Service, The Library of Congress.

Tumlinson, A., Reester, H., & Missmar, R. (2003). *Limitations in Medicare managed care options for integration with Medicaid.* Lawrenceville, NJ: Center for Health Care Strategies.

U.S. General Accounting Office. (1995). *Medicaid: Restructuring approaches leave many questions.* Washington, DC: GAO, Pub No. GAO/HEHS-95-103.

Verdier, J., Gold, M., & Davis, S. (2008). *Do we know if Medicare Advantage special needs plans are special?* Menlo Park, CA: Henry J. Kaiser Family Foundation.

Walsh, E. G., & Clark, W. D. (2002). Managed care and dually eligible beneficiaries: Challenges in coordination. *Health Care Financing Review, 24*(1), 63–82.

Walsh, E. G., Freiman, M., Haber, S., Bragg, A., Ouslander, J., & Wiener, J. M. (2010). *Cost drivers for dually eligible beneficiaries: Potentially avoidable hospitalizations from nursing facility, skilled nursing facility, and home and community-based services waiver programs.* Washington, DC: Final Task 2 Report, CMS Contract No. HHSM-500-2005-00029I.

Weissert, W. G., Lesnick, T., Musliner, M., & Foley, K. A. (1997). Cost savings from home and community-based services: Arizona's capitated Medicaid long-term care program. *Journal of Health Politics, Policy, and Law, 22*(6), 1329–1357.

White, A. J., Abel, Y., & Kidder, D. (2000). *A comparison of the PACE capitation rates to projected costs in the first year of enrollment: Final report.* Cambridge, MA: Report Prepared for HCFA by Abt Associates, Inc.

Medicare and the Affordable Care Act

MARILYN MOON, PhD
Senior Vice President, American Institutes for Research,
Silver Spring, Maryland, USA

The recently enacted Patient Protection and Affordable Care Act made modest changes to improve Medicare and obtained a substantial share of funding for the Act's broader reforms from future spending reductions in the program. Drug benefits and preventive services were improved. While painful, the spending reductions will have only moderate impacts on beneficiaries and should help achieve the goals of health care reform: encouraging better primary and preventive care, making providers conscious of finding ways to increase the productivity of care delivered and changing the relative levels of payment across certain providers. Additional costs to beneficiaries will arise from changes in private plan payments and increasing income-related premiums.

INTRODUCTION

While much of the focus of the health reform legislation passed in 2010 was on expanding coverage to the younger-than-65 population, a number of changes will affect older Americans as well. And although much of this issue is focusing on long-term care, it is also important to examine other areas of the Patient Protection and Affordable Care Act (ACA) that affect seniors and disabled Medicare beneficiaries.[1] The ACA made modest changes to improve the Medicare program and obtained a substantial share of revenue to pay for new benefits provided by the ACA from slowing spending on Medicare over time. Even if there were no issues specific to Medicare, seniors have a stake in an affordable health care system that works for everyone.

In this article, I examine provisions that both improve Medicare benefits and that slow the rate of growth in payments to doctors, hospitals, and other providers. On balance, most of the changes focus on the appropriate areas for improvement in Medicare, although they do not go far enough to resolve the problems of Medicare's inadequacies. Benefit improvements include:

- Better protection against the costs of prescription drugs
- Better coverage of preventive and other services
- Modestly improved access to primary care physicians
- Minor improvements for the Medicare low-income population

Key changes that will reduce Medicare spending include:

- Payment reform for Medicare Advantage
- Reductions in annual payment growth for hospitals and other non-physician providers
- Expansions in beneficiary premiums for those with higher incomes
- Creation of an independent commission to restrain spending growth over time

It is important to put these proposed changes into an appropriate context. Effective health reform can substantially improve our heath care system, even if it falls short of everyone's "ideal." Similarly, changes in Medicare can improve its effectiveness—even those designed to achieve savings. It is also important to keep in mind what would happen to the health care system and Medicare in the absence of the ACA. Regardless of whether health care reform legislation had passed, pressures for holding down costs would continue—both for Medicare and for private insurance as taxpayers and employers, respectively, found the rate of growth of spending to be an increasingly untenable burden. Both Medicare and health care spending as a whole have grown faster than gross domestic product (GDP) for most of the past 46 years. As a result, health care spending continues to grow as a share of the overall economy; at some point this share will begin to crowd out other desired spending. If the rate of health care spending averages 2.5% above GDP in the future, federal outlays would rise from 18.4% of GDP in 2007 to 28.5% in 2050 (Aaron, 2007).

IMPROVED MEDICARE BENEFITS

The expansions enacted for Medicare beneficiaries address some of the well-known gaps in benefits and assure that access to care will be improved over time. These are important first steps toward a more comprehensive benefit package for this critical group of the U.S. population, but they still leave Medicare less comprehensive than the coverage that many Americans with employer-sponsored insurance have.

Closing the Gap in Drug Coverage and Other Part D Changes

When the prescription drug benefit under Medicare became law in 2003, there was insufficient funding to offer a fully comprehensive benefit, given the constraints that federal policymakers agreed to impose on spending. President Bush and the Congress limited subsidies to a predetermined amount—which were stretched to cover both catastrophic expenses and enough basic coverage to encourage relatively healthy people to sign up for the benefit (Zhang, Donohue, Newhouse, & Lave, 2009). That left a gap in coverage or "donut hole" as it has come to be called. In 2011, the gap in coverage occurred for those beneficiaries with annual expenses over $2,840 (Board of Trustees, 2011). At that point, insurance protection ceased until affected beneficiaries spent $7,390 on drugs or a total of $4,550 out-of-pocket. After that, catastrophic protection—covering 95% of the cost of drugs—began. For many Medicare beneficiaries, this is an important gap in coverage.

Evidence shows that enrollees in Part D plans who have chronic conditions and take multiple medications each day are likely to fall into the donut hole at some time during the year. It has been estimated that about 3.4 million enrollees in Part D (about 14% of all enrollees) enter the coverage gap in any given year (Kaiser Family Foundation, 2009a). A number of these beneficiaries stop taking at least some of their drugs during this period. Failure to take medications daily leaves beneficiaries at risk for poorer health and increased health expenditures over time (Zhang et al., 2009). While private insurers could offer coverage for these expenses in the gap, they receive no government subsidy so very few now do so, with the exception that some plans cover inexpensive, generic drugs. In fact, since the program began in 2006, fewer plans each year offer gap coverage; there has been a race to the minimum by insurers, resulting in lower premiums but also less comprehensive benefits (Kaiser Family Foundation, 2011b).

In 2010, the ACA provided each Medicare beneficiary reaching the donut hole a $250 payment to help defray medication costs. Beginning in 2011, a 50% discount on the cost of brand name drugs is being given to each beneficiary who falls into the donut hole, but the full cost of those drugs counts toward the annual out-of-pocket spending that must be met before catastrophic protections begin. Consequently, people reach the catastrophic protection level with lower actual out-of-pocket spending than in the past. This approach effectively helps to close the gap in coverage over time. The federal government then will gradually increase the amount covered until the insurance protection reaches 75% of the costs of prescriptions (the same protection now guaranteed before reaching the donut hole); the phase-in period will take 11 years (Kaiser Family Foundation, 2010b). To eliminate the donut hole immediately would have required spending of about $137 billion over 10 years (Congressional Budget Office, 2010) and was deemed to add too much to the costs of reform in the negotiations over how to keep the costs of the ACA below $1 trillion. Just as with the earlier drug legislation, many elements of the ACA were chosen to achieve the goal of meeting specific budget targets. This more than sound policy analysis often dictated the specifics of the legislation (Newhouse, 2010).

The ACA also provides some important consumer protections, for example, limiting how much a plan can change the drugs on the formulary during the year, improving the appeals process, and providing more oversight and tracking of the program. While these changes do not fully resolve the problems facing beneficiaries from an inadequate drug benefit that can raise costs to beneficiaries and/or lower use of needed medications (Zhang et al., 2009), the ACA will represent a substantial improvement over time.

Better Coverage for Preventive and Other Services

Before 2010, beneficiaries were required to pay the Part B deductible and coinsurance on preventive services, potentially discouraging individuals from using these services (Kaplan, 2011). The ACA eliminated these charges, reducing what beneficiaries must pay for those preventive services deemed to meet a rating of effectiveness by the U.S. Preventive Services Task Force. In addition, the new law adds a yearly wellness visit with no coinsurance requirement. In the past, such visits were only available in the year that the beneficiary entered the Medicare program. More generous coverage of preventive services following implementation of the ACA should lower premiums for supplemental Medigap coverage over time as the savings from these changes reduce the costs to insurers.

Another service improvement that was in the House bill but omitted by the final legislation was for consultations for advanced care planning (Parsons & Zajac, 2009). This is the source of the infamous claims about a "death panel" requirement in the legislation. For a number of years, analysts and researchers have argued that health care professionals do not do a very good job of helping patients sort out their options when they are facing challenges such as a terminal illness (Moon, 2006). The House version of the bill would have provided additional support services, offering patients who wished to discuss such issues an opportunity to do so. More importantly, there would have been no mandatory aspect to this newly covered benefit. This provision would have been an expansion of services added in 2003 without controversy (Parsons & Zajac, 2009).

Also missing from the legislation was an upper bound on cost-sharing liability. This is a crucial benefit found in most employer-provided insurance but missing from Medicare. It is a deficiency in coverage that makes purchase of supplemental coverage an important additional cost for beneficiaries who want to protect themselves from unlimited exposure to out-of-pocket costs (Moon, 2006).

Payment Reform and Better Access to Physicians

For a number of years, physicians have faced the prospect of substantial cuts in Medicare payments each year because of a flaw in the annual payment update formula. This problem keeps being put off temporarily, but the underlying requirement has not changed. Thus, each year the potential cut in payments grows larger. It was scheduled to be about 23% in 2010 and the House bill would have tackled this problem permanently (Sisko et al., 2010). It is, however, very expensive to do and hence was not in the more restricted Senate version of health reform that became law in 2010. The only adjustment included in the ACA was a temporary fix, increasing payments by 0.5% in 2010; another temporary fix has since been passed by Congress, holding off any payment cuts in 2011 (Foster, 2010). A more permanent fix was promised but is still uncertain, so this issue remains a looming problem facing the Medicare program over time (Medicare Payment Advisory Commission [MedPAC], 2011). Failure to deal directly with this issue is a disappointing aspect of health reform, particularly since it was recognized as a major problem with Medicare but allowed to remain unaddressed.

The new law does, however, recognize the importance of improving payments for office visits by increasing payments by 10% for primary care doctors who receive at least 60% of their revenues from these services. Over time, payments for treatments by specialists in Medicare have grown relative to office visits even as interest in promoting primary care has become an accepted policy goal (MedPAC, 2011). This increase in payments, both for office visits and for physicians working in health professional shortage areas, will be paid for by reducing payments for other physician services (Kaiser Family Foundation, 2010b). When combined with a more permanent fix for the update factor, these changes should improve payments for primary care physicians who are in increasingly short supply but who are critical for implementing many of the changes anticipated in redirecting the way that care is delivered in the United States. Without the permanent fix, however, this change has been largely overlooked as physicians must each year worry about a larger cut in their fees.

Minor Improvements in Low-Income Protections

Another important area often identified for improving Medicare is in protections for low-income beneficiaries. The traditional Medicaid program is the most comprehensive source of protection, but in many states, it does not even cover all those below the poverty threshold. Other, more limited protections include Medicaid payment of Medicare cost sharing and premiums for those up to 135% of the federal poverty level (FPL) and the low-income subsidy program under the Part D drug benefit that extends up to 150% of the FPL. The maximum of 150% of the FPL—about $16,500 in income for an individual in 2011—still leaves many beneficiaries with very high cost-sharing burdens (Kaiser Family Foundation, 2011c). Proposed expansions of the Part D subsidy did not make it into the final legislation, however. The one change that was included waives coinsurance and deductibles under Part D for non-institutionalized individuals eligible for both Medicare and Medicaid—the so-called dually eligible. Since many dually eligible had more generous benefits when they received drug coverage under Medicaid than at present under Medicare Part D (Commonwealth Fund, 2007), this is an important restoration of protection that could help lower their burdens. Other improvements to expand eligibility for low-income protections did not take place. Consequently, the most generous protections remain limited to beneficiaries with incomes below 150% of the FPL.

MEDICARE SAVINGS PROPOSALS

Changes to Medicare payment served as a major source of financing health reform's benefits for the younger-than-65 population in the ACA. Critics have characterized these proposals as "starving" the Medicare program and threatening care. In fact, this was a major criticism of ACA leveled by Republicans in the 2010 elections, although very little analysis was offered regarding these claims. In actuality, most of the changes focus on payments to providers of care and not coverage or access. The major concern for beneficiaries is whether these cuts will reduce the willingness of providers to continue serving Medicare beneficiaries. These reductions are proportionately lower than reductions that have been made in the program several times over the years (Kaiser Family Foundation, 2009b) and—in contrast to past payment reductions—will be offset by improved revenues to providers from expanded coverage for the younger population (Newhouse, 2010).

Most of the savings described below will not have a direct impact on beneficiaries, with two important exceptions. First, the Medicare Advantage program, where beneficiaries may choose to get their care from a private plan option, will be subject to substantial reductions in levels of payment that may affect benefits offered to individuals. Second, higher-income beneficiaries are now subjected to an expansion in the income-related premium in Part B and to a new income-related premium in Part D, increasing their out-of-pocket costs (Kaplan, 2011).

Payment Reform for Medicare Advantage

Legislation in 2003 established what are now regarded to be "excess" payments to the Medicare Advantage program (MedPAC, 2009). The goal in providing extra payments after 2003 was to encourage private plans to offer options to Medicare beneficiaries by enticing them with incentive payments. Presumably, this excess should have gone away once plans opted to participate in Medicare Advantage, resulting in lower payments over time (Gold, 2008). But, in 2009, these payments still averaged 14% above what it would cost to provide Medicare coverage in the traditional fee-for-service portion of the program (MedPAC, 2010). Despite a bidding process, plans continued to cost the Medicare program more and hence have raised Part B premiums for those not in private plans since the higher costs to Medicare from these plans are included when premiums are calculated as 25% of Medicare costs. As a consequence, this has created serious inequities between those in private plans and those remaining in traditional Medicare.

Plans receiving overpayments have often offered additional services to their enrollees. This was usually in the form of lower-cost prescription drug plans or vision and dental services. Some of the coinsurance and deductibles required are lower than those contained in traditional Medicare. But overall, beneficiaries receive only a portion of the "excess subsidy" that is provided by Medicare to private plans (Commonwealth Fund, 2011). As payments to Medicare Advantage plans are reduced over time in response to the ACA, some of these extra services will likely be reduced or eliminated or premiums to enroll in the private plans will rise. Many private plans have complained that this will hurt their enrollees, and some have threatened to pull out of the program. As of fall 2011, however, few plans have withdrawn (Commonwealth Fund, 2011).

How should such changes be viewed? In some ways, the proposal is analogous to the closing of a tax loophole where people who previously benefited now must pay taxes comparable to those like themselves but who did not have access to (or for other reasons chose not to use) the loophole. The loss of these windfall gains will undoubtedly be painful for some beneficiaries but will not affect the bulk of Medicare recipients. In 2009, more than 75% of Medicare beneficiaries were in the traditional part of Medicare and hence did not have access to any windfall benefits (MedPAC, 2010). Moreover, even for those in Medicare Advantage, not all receive extra benefits. For example, private fee-for-service plans provide few extra benefits, and because some of them offer different combinations of cost sharing, beneficiaries may pay even more out of pocket (Gold, 2008). While many beneficiaries live in areas where such private plans exist, they choose not to enroll, often because they have multiple doctors on whom they rely and who do not participate in the private plans (Commonwealth Fund, 2011).

Others may live in areas where plans have not offered many extra benefits and will see little change.

Moreover, the legislation is not punitive. Only modest changes are being made in 2011, and the full change will not be complete until 2015. Early evidence suggests that enrollment has not dropped off as much as was projected by either formal estimates or the plans themselves (Kaiser Family Foundation, 2011d). Further, plans that demonstrate excellence will be offered bonuses that will soften the blow of the changes. In particular, plans that achieve certain performance goals will be provided with additional payments per enrollee. In 2012, a large majority of plans are scheduled to receive such bonuses (Kaiser Family Foundation, 2011a). The ultimate goal is to offer payments to private plans equivalent to what beneficiaries would cost the traditional fee-for-service portion of the program had they not enrolled in Medicare Advantage. Total savings have been estimated at $135 billion over 10 years (see Table 1; Congressional Budget Office, 2010).

Finally, a number of protections for consumers have been added that will improve assurances that when beneficiaries do enroll in Medicare Advantage, the plan will be one that meets the promises it makes. Marketing reforms and greater oversight on issues such as cost sharing requirements and medical loss ratios (to ensure that plans are paying out a substantial share of their premiums in benefits) should improve the care that individuals receive under these plans.

Income-Related Beneficiary Premiums

The ACA increases the income-related premium for Part B services and adds a new income-related premium to Part D that effectively reduces the subsidy now offered under the drug benefit. Together these changes are projected

TABLE 1 Dollar Savings From Major Medicare Changes

Provisions	2010–2014	2010–2019
Payment Adjustment for Conditions Acquired in Hospitals	$0.0	$−1.4
Establishment of Center for Medicare and Medicaid Innovation	0.7	−1.3
Medicare Shared Savings Program	−0.5	−4.9
Hospital Readmissions Reduction Program	−0.5	−7.1
Payment Adjustments for Home Health Care	−4.2	−39.7
Medicare Disproportionate Share Hospital Payments	0.0	−22.1
Equipment Utilization Factor for Advanced Imaging Services	−0.9	−2.3
Medicare Advantage Payments	−30.3	−135.6
Reducing Part D Premium Subsidy for High-Income Beneficiaries	−2.4	−10.7
Revision of Certain Market Basket Updates	−23.7	−156.6
Temporary Adjustment to the Calculation of Part B Premiums	−7.5	−25.0
Independent Payment Advisory Board	0.0	−15.5

Note. Source: Congressional Budget Office, 2010.

to raise an additional $36 billion in new revenues (Congressional Budget Office, 2010). Normally, the threshold at which beneficiaries begin to pay the income-related premium rises each year as incomes rise, holding the share of beneficiaries subject to the additional premium relatively constant. Under ACA, this threshold is frozen from 2011 to 2019. Thus, those who have incomes above $85,000 for singles and $170,000 for couples will continue to be subject to the tax for a number of years, rather than seeing these thresholds rise as the cost of living goes up. This will mean that more and more beneficiaries will be subject to the higher, income-related premium each year, reaching 3.5 million by 2019 (Kaiser Family Foundation, 2010a).

The new Part D income-related premium has been established to operate in much the same way as that for Part B, effectively increasing the cost of purchasing insurance on those whose incomes are above the threshold. Unlike Part B where most beneficiaries enroll, Part D is less likely to be used by high-income beneficiaries who often have employer-provided retiree coverage; hence, they are less likely to be in Part D in the first place (Kaiser Family Foundation, 2011b). While the number of beneficiaries affected by changes to the Part B and Part D premiums will be small, the number of people subject to higher premiums will rise while the costs of Medicare to those who pay those premiums will increase considerably. There is some concern that these costs may discourage participation in Parts B and D over time and hence undercut some of the strong support that currently exists for the program (Kaplan, 2011).

Reducing Medicare Payment Growth

The largest source of funding for health reform will come from reductions in payments for many Medicare program benefits, including skilled nursing care, home health benefits, and outpatient hospital services as compared to their projected levels before passage of the ACA (Foster, 2010). This generally means that the rate of growth of payments is projected to be slower than the law currently dictates and in line with similar changes made over the past several decades. Critical to evaluating these payment changes is whether they are consistent with providers' ability to improve efficiency in service delivery or whether they will threaten access to or quality of care, especially relative to non-Medicare patients. But just as critical is whether these changes would have been made at some point anyway: Are they necessary for the health of the Medicare program that continues to be under financial pressure? Will they be consistent with how the rest of the health care system pays providers? Furthermore, regardless of the potential desirability of such changes, the Medicare actuary has suggested that the level of cuts anticipated may be difficult to sustain over time (Foster, 2010). This dynamic has played out previously. While the Balanced Budget Act of 1997 made substantial reductions in skilled nursing facility and home health agency payments, some reductions were given back through subsequent legislation after the adverse implications for providers' financial well-being materialized.

The largest changes that result in savings will have an across-the-board effect on services provided in Part A institutions (all types of hospitals, skilled nursing facilities, hospice care) by changing the market basket adjustment that is used each year to determine how much payment rates will increase over the preceding year. The adjustments under the ACA were justified as reflecting expected productivity increases that should allow facilities to provide care without having to receive a full market basket update. These savings are estimated to be about $116 billion—less than 5% of the total payments that were projected to go to these services (under Part A of Medicare) over the next 10 years. In addition, payments will be frozen for a year for skilled nursing facilities and inpatient rehabilitation facility payments, largely because of analyses that have indicated that these payments are sufficient to retain access to care (MedPAC, 2010). In fact, over time such services have grown rapidly, indicating providers' willingness to offer such care. Home health is a spectacular example, having grown by 71% between 2005 and 2010 (Board of Trustees, 2011).

Reductions in Part B service payments other than those for physician services are also included in the ACA. Similar changes in annual updates to account for productivity improvements will be made for outpatient facilities, laboratory services, and some durable medical equipment. This will add another $40 billion in savings on the Part B side of Medicare. The total from changes to the market basket update is thus over $156 billion (Congressional Budget Office, 2010). Will reductions in payments to Part A and B providers harm access to care or quality for Medicare patients? These same types of adjustments have been used extensively in the past, particularly in the 1980s and early 1990s (Kaiser Family Foundation, 2009b). Providers have traditionally responded rapidly to Medicare changes. In response to payment changes in the early 1980s, for example, hospitals reduced their lengths of stay enormously (Moon, 2006).

More recently, the Balanced Budget Act of 1997 constrained growth rates in hospital payments by reducing the annual payment increases for hospitals. Prices were frozen in 1998 and then constrained in growth for the next 4 years. These savings were expected to slow hospital spending by about $33 billion or about 8% of expected spending over 5 years. But savings turned out to be even larger. Within 3 years, the expected insolvency date for the Medicare Part A trust fund, which covers inpatient hospital care, was extended from 4 to 25 years. While some later adjustments were made to soften the impact, hospitals nevertheless were able to achieve enough productivity increases that Medicare has remained a reasonable payer from the facilities' vantage point (MedPAC, 2009).

After years of consistently reducing the rate of growth of payments as a mechanism for holding down costs, Medicare benefits have not had such constraints applied for the last 6 years, leaving open the opportunity for achieving savings now. Hospitals may challenge reductions in payment updates with claims that they lose money from Medicare. Medicare payment rates are indeed below those of private payers. But for about two-thirds of all hospitals, Medicare's payments exceed the cost of care (MedPAC, 2010). Moreover, MedPAC has found that the hospitals that lost money on Medicare are in areas where private insurers are not pressuring them to reduce costs. Medicare payments exceed costs where hospitals are pressured to be more efficient. Efficient hospitals can be role models for the rest (MedPAC, 2009).

Skilled nursing facilities and other specialty facilities have considerable room for efficiencies and show no signs of cutting access to Medicare patients (MedPAC, 2010). In the past, these institutions have done an excellent job of lobbying for adjustments when necessary, and MedPAC and others monitor care to determine whether quality or access issues arise.

A number of other reforms to the payment systems are also part of ACA; in particular, savings would be obtained from changing the way in which the home health program operates. Home health agencies have done very well under the episode-based payment system established a few years ago, likely helping to explain why the number of providers has grown rapidly over time (MedPAC, 2010). Since agencies are paid on an episode basis, they may benefit while *not* increasing access to services for beneficiaries. This is an area where reform could achieve savings and actually help beneficiaries receive more appropriate levels of care. The ACA also seeks to achieve savings from changing current incentives to providers in ways that will improve the quality of care. For example, the Congressional Budget Office (2010) estimates that over $19 billion can be saved by reducing payments to hospitals that have high readmissions in areas that were preventable. The goal is to get hospitals to take extra precautions to assure that patients do not have to return unnecessarily. Savings from this source should be viewed as an improvement in care for beneficiaries.

Further, the ACA established a Patient-Centered Outcomes Research Institute to encourage study about how well various alternative drugs or treatments work as compared to each other. Such analyses are important since very little scientific evidence of what actually works well in practice exists, and many analysts believe that this is a critical effort for assuring reasonable costs in the future (Newhouse, 2010). While there has been some concern expressed over such work leading to the denial of care, the legislation is quite restrictive in terms of how it could be used. Furthermore, better analysis and information on what works is an important tool in a world in which we must be conscious of the costs of care. When studies indicate that care is ineffective or even harmful, quality of care can be improved by doing *less*.

The ACA also created a Center for Innovation in Medicare and Medicaid to explore issues in payment and delivery system reforms. Historically, the private sector has followed Medicare's lead in instituting payment reforms (Moon, 2006). In combination with requirements for demonstrations on the medical home and other activities, the push for new ideas and approaches to health care—and the resources to support those innovations—could also generate positive outcomes for everyone (Newhouse, 2010). To the extent that these involve administrative changes and regulations, reforms could be implemented without requiring further Congressional approval.

Along with concerns about access and quality, assessing proposed savings must take into account the near-universal agreement that something must be done to rein in the costs of health care spending over time—not just for Medicare but for the entire health care system (Aaron, 2007; Newhouse, 2010). Health care analysts have consistently argued that it is difficult to expect systemic reforms to be introduced in only one part of the system. Even though Medicare is a large and crucial payer of services, many changes would work best if instituted across the board. For example, adoption of evidence-based guidelines and treatment approaches need to be universal, and payment changes that affect only one payer have the potential for shifting of costs onto others.

Independent Payment Advisory Board

To assure continued savings in Medicare over time, the ACA establishes a 15-member Medicare commission that would operate independently to guarantee that Medicare spending would not grow excessively over time. The Independent Payment Advisory Board, which begins operations in 2018, will be tasked with recommending Medicare changes to hold the rate of growth of spending to GDP per capita plus 1% in 2019 and beyond. The restrictions envisioned from the Independent Payment Advisory Board have resulted in criticism from a broad range of policymakers, usually centered on the concern that the need to meet certain targets will lead to rationing of care. While it is precluded from changing benefits or cost sharing requirements, the Independent Payment Advisory Board could, however, be problematic for beneficiaries. Setting absolute growth targets may fail to offer the flexibility that might be needed in future years. For example, since the allowed growth rate would be tied to GDP, what would happen in case of another severe recession such as we have been experiencing? The need for health care does not fall just because of a financial crisis. Further, true innovations that can lower costs over time can increase costs in the short run. And establishing constraints only on Medicare may move the program away from the mainstream of care offered to others. Finally, if it gets harder to find savings from payment and other reforms, will the rules excluding changes in benefits or cost sharing be eased? It is important to assure that Medicare continues to be in the mainstream of health care delivery and not be inordinately singled out for change in order to avoid the risk of harming beneficiaries' access to care.

CONCLUSION

The changes legislated for the Medicare program include a combination of expansions and reductions in payments and modest improvements in coverage. On the whole, these changes are designed to improve the program and achieve the goals of health care reform: encouraging better primary and preventive care, making providers conscious of finding ways to increase the productivity of care delivered, and rebalancing payment levels where they are either too high or too low. The improvements are modest but in line with the fiscal limits that Congress has prescribed overall for health care reform. It is the case that the Medicare program is being subjected to limits on spending growth in order to help fund care for younger populations, raising legitimate questions about whether care for the younger-than-65 population should largely be funded by changes that will have some potential negative consequences on Medicare providers and beneficiaries. Nonetheless, the claims that Medicare will be severely undermined and that seniors will be harmed have been overstated. Moreover, these very same reductions in payments would likely have been prominent options under discussion for the deficit reduction efforts that are likely to be part of the debate on Medicare's future if they were not already part of the new health legislation. The payment slowdown and other changes will extend the life of the Medicare Part A trust fund by 12 years, helping to put the program on stronger financial footing (Mussey, 2010).

It is also important to consider what these changes might mean for long-term care and those who need such services. Greater restrictions on home health services and skilled nursing care are likely to have some negative effects on access. Other changes, however, might be more positive. Encouraging better coordination of care from medical homes or accountable care organizations, for example, might lead to better integration of acute and long-term care services. But it will take some time for investment in innovations to generate results that could improve care. Further, better coverage of the younger-than-65 population and expansion in preventive services in Medicare could also contribute further to improvements in health status and reduced need for long-term care over time. That is, studies indicate that those who enter Medicare with periods of no insurance coverage prior to eligibility have substantially higher rates of spending under Medicare for several years (McWilliams, Meara, Zaslavsky, & Ayanian, 2007).

Finally, while it is tempting to ask who wins or loses in Medicare, we all have a stake in an improved health care system that meets the needs of all Americans. For example, reducing the use of ineffective tests or procedures can both save costs and avoid potential problems from the unnecessary care that results (Pearson & Bach, 2010). Healthier Americans will contribute more to society, bolster our ability to afford care, and lower the costs to Medicare that now arise when people who have had poor access to care place avoidable burdens on the Medicare program once they do enroll. The health care system will change over time; the goal is to make those changes apply fairly and reasonably for all Americans, including those covered by Medicare.

NOTE

1. For the specific aspects of the legislation, see the Patient Protection and Affordable Care Act, *Pub. L. No. 111–148, 124 Stat. 119* (2010). In addition, a good description can also be found in materials from the Kaiser Family Foundation at KaiserFamilyFoundation.org. Some of them are specifically referenced here. Details on the dollar amounts of the components of the legislation come from the Congressional Budget Office (2010).

REFERENCES

Aaron, H. (2007). Budget crisis, entitlement crisis, health care financing problem—which is it? *Health Affairs, 26*(6), 1622–1635.

Board of Trustees. (2011). *2011 annual report of the Boards of Trustees of the Federal Hospital Insurance and Federal Supplementary Medical Insurance Trust Funds.* Baltimore, MD: Center for Medicare and Medicaid Services.

Commonwealth Fund. (2007). *Improving the Medicare Part D Program for the most vulnerable beneficiaries.* New York, NY: The Commonwealth Fund, Pub. No. 1031. May.

Commonwealth Fund. (2011). *Medicare Advantage in the era of health reform: Progress in leveling the playing field.* New York, NY: The Commonwealth Fund, Pub. No. 1491. March.

Congressional Budget Office. (2009). *Letter to Senator Max Baucus,* October 7, 2009.

Congressional Budget Office. (2010). *Selected CBO publications related to health care legislation, 2009–2010.* Washington, DC: GPO. December.

Foster, R. (2010). *Estimated financial effects of the Patient Protection and Affordable Care Act, as passed by the Senate on December 24, 2009.* Baltimore, MD: Office of the Actuary, Centers for Medicare and Medicaid Services. January 8, Memorandum.

Gold, M. (2008). Medicare's private plans: A report card on Medicare Advantage. *Health Affairs, 28*(1), w41–w54.

Kaplan, R. (2011). Analyzing the impact of the new health care reform legislation on older Americans. *The Elder Law Journal, 18*(2), 213–245.

Kaiser Family Foundation. (2009a). *Tracking Medicare health and prescription drug plans.* Monthly Report for July.

Kaiser Family Foundation. (2009b). *Medicare savings in perspective: A comparison of 2009 health reform legislation and other laws in the last 15 years.* Focus on Health Reform, December.

Kaiser Family Foundation. (2010a). *Income-relating Medicare Part B and Part D premiums: How many Medicare beneficiaries will be affected?* December, Issue Brief.

Kaiser Family Foundation. (2010b). *Summary of key changes to Medicare in 2010 health reform law*. Publication 7948-02. Retrieved from http://www.Kaiser Family Foundation.org

Kaiser Family Foundation. (2011a). *Medicare Advantage Plan star ratings and bonus payments in 2012*. November, Data Brief.

Kaiser Family Foundation. (2011b). *Analysis of Medicare prescription drug plans in 2011 and key trends since 2006*. September, Issue Brief.

Kaiser Family Foundation. (2011c). *Health care on a budget: The financial burden of health spending by Medicare households*. June, Data Spotlight.

Kaiser Family Foundation. (2011d). *Tracking Medicare health and prescription drug plans*. Monthly Report for January.

Medicare Payment Advisory Commission (MedPAC). (2009). *Report to Congress: Medicare payment policy*. Washington, DC: MedPAC, March.

Medicare Payment Advisory Commission (MedPAC). (2010). *Report to Congress: Medicare payment policy*. Washington, DC: MedPAC, March.

Medicare Payment Advisory Commission (MedPAC). (2011). *Report to Congress: Medicare payment policy*. Washington, DC: MedPAC, March.

McWilliams, J. M., Meara, E., Zaslavsky, A., & Ayanian, J. (2007). Use of health services by previously uninsured Medicare beneficiaries. *New England Journal of Medicine, 357*(2), 143–153.

Moon, M. (2006). *Medicare: A policy primer*. Washington, DC: Urban Institute Press.

Mussey, S. (2010). *Estimated effects of the Patient Protection and Affordable Care Act, as passed by the Senate on the year of exhaustion for the Part A trust fund, Part B premiums, and Part A and Part B coinsurance amounts*. Baltimore, MD: Office of the Actuary, Centers for Medicare and Medicaid Services. Memorandum, January 8.

Newhouse, Joseph. (2010). Assessing health reform's impact on four key groups of Americans. *Health Affairs, 29*(9), 1714–1724.

Parsons, C., & Zajac, A. (2009). Fight looms over Medicare Advantage, which Obama Administration wants to trim. *Los Angeles Times*, August 19.

Pearson, S., & Bach, P. (2010). How Medicare could use comparative effectiveness research in deciding on new coverage and reimbursement. *Health Affairs, 29*(10), 1796–1804.

Sisko, A., Truffer, C., Keehan, S., Posal, J., Kent Clemens, M., & Andrew Madison, A. (2010). National health spending projections: The estimated impact of reform through 2019. *Health Affairs, 29*(10), 1933–1941.

Zhang, Y., Donohue, J., Newhouse, J., & Lave, J. (2009). The effects of the coverage gap on drug spending: A closer look at Medicare Part D. *Health Affairs, 28*(2), w317–w325.

CONCLUSION

The Affordable Care Act, Long-Term Care, and Elders: Two Steps Forward, One Step Back

PAMELA NADASH, PhD

Assistant Professor of Gerontology, and Fellow, Gerontology Institute,
University of Massachusetts Boston, Boston, Massachusetts, USA

EDWARD ALAN MILLER, PhD, MPA

Associate Professor of Gerontology and Public Policy, and Fellow,
Gerontology Institute, University of Massachusetts Boston, Boston,
Massachusetts, USA

This essay places the essays in this volume in the context of policy development for health- and long-term care (LTC), by positioning the Patient Protection and Affordable Care Act (ACA) of 2010 within the American tradition of incrementalism. It discusses how most of the law's provisions constitute incremental advances in existing strategies and fail to address the fundamental and structural issues that prevent genuine advancement in this policy area. Instead, we see a continuation of current strategies for improving services for older people, some of which nonetheless hold considerable promise, including strategies to expand home- and community-based care, improve and expand the long-term care workforce, address prevailing deficiencies in nursing home quality, and better coordinate care received by LTC recipients and other frail and disabled individuals. The primary exception to this, the Community Living Assistance Services and Supports (CLASS) Act, is unlikely to be implemented in its existing form; however, debate over its design reveals the fundamental lack of agreement in the American policy community about the appropriate role of government in long-term care. Ultimately, the impact of the ACA will be mediated by the extent to which both the federal and state governments opt to invest in it, through funding, implementing, and enforcing the ACA's provisions.

The essays in this volume demonstrate how the Patient Protection and Affordable Care Act (ACA) of 2010 continues the great American tradition of incrementalism. Even within this landmark piece of legislation, which took a big step forward by promoting universal health insurance coverage, we see, as in other policy areas, a reliance on small steps–policies that continue along well-trod paths (Tuohy, 2011). Although this is unsurprising, given the current political environment, it also means that the legislation fails to address some of the fundamental flaws of our health, and particularly long-term care (LTC), systems. Perhaps the most salient exception to this incrementalist model was the Community Living Assistance Services and Supports (CLASS) Act; an effort to expand access to LTC financing in the U.S. However Because of concerns about program solvency the Obama administration suspended implementation of CLASS in October 2011; as such, the program is unlikely to be implemented in its existing form, if at all (Department of Health and Human Services, 2011). Instead, the ACA continues current strategies for improving services for older people, some of which nonetheless hold considerable promise, including strategies to expand home- and community-based care, improve and expand the LTC workforce, address prevailing deficiencies in nursing home quality, and better coordinate care received by LTC recipients and other frail and disabled individuals. Ultimately, the impact of the ACA's LTC provisions will be mediated by the extent to which the government opts to invest in these strategies, through funding, implementing, and enforcing the changes made.

The bulk of this volume is devoted to the ACA's LTC initiatives, which, overall, are consistent with the history of LTC policy in the United States. Development of a coherent approach to LTC has been a long struggle (Ogden & Adams, 2008; Smith & Feng, 2010; Yee, 2001), one which is far from complete. The marginal position of LTC in the social safety net was marked as early as the Medicare design process, when it was quickly dropped as a potential coverage option and relegated to the hastily-introduced Medicaid program, where the breadth and quality of coverage were left mainly to the states (Marmor, 2000). The emergence of Medicaid as the primary payer (and the subsequent use of nursing homes as the primary venue for care, resulting from the inclusion of nursing home care as a required service under the program) was an unintended consequence of this decision (Smith & Feng 2010). This poorly thought out approach to LTC policymaking is only too typical of an issue area that, outside of a few noteworthy examples, has lacked strong legislative advocates (as Hawes notes, in her piece: Gleckman, 2011)–a lack that no doubt mirrors the low level of public awareness of this issue (Mature Market Institute, 2009).

Low public awareness has further consequences: most importantly, despite the growing number of Americans affected by the need for LTC—whether as service recipients or caregivers—the general public is poorly prepared for the future. When pressed, many wrongly think that LTC is covered by Medicare; that their family members will provide sufficient care; or that they are low risk; the cost of long-term care insurance (LTCI) plans is also a major deterrent (LifePlans, Inc., 2007; Mature Market Institute, 2009). Thus, many people fail to take the necessity of planning for their LTC needs seriously, a failure reinforced by competing messages regarding the need to save for retirement and plan for future healthcare expenses.

The inability to develop a coherent federal approach to the issue has also been influenced by the lack of consensus regarding what exactly that federal role should be. Many feel that LTC should be a family and individual responsibility and, consequently, that this area is better suited to private sector solutions–for the non-poor, at least (Moses, 2005, Yee, 2001). However, efforts to encourage market-based solutions appear to have had little impact; these mainly focus on encouraging people to buy private long-term care insurance (LTCI), although there is intermittent discussion of other financial vehicles to cover the cost of LTC (Ahlstrom, Tumlinson & Lambrew, 2004;

Feder, Komisar & Friedland, 2007; Murtaugh, Spillman & Warshawsky, 2001). Early moves in this area included a 1997 decision to make certain LTCI plans tax-deductible and a 2000 decision to establish LTCI as a benefit for federal employees. Another effort has been the ongoing "Own Your Future" campaign, launched in 2005, where various government departments have worked with individual states to roll out information campaigns encouraging people to plan for future LTC needs. Despite efforts such as these, the purchase of LTCI has remained limited to a small proportion of the population, a trend largely explained by the high cost of policies. This suggests that government-led efforts to promote private sector solutions in this area are failing to achieve one of government's primary goals: reducing dependence on public programs.

The most significant federal initiative to increase LTCI coverage has been the LTC Partnership Programs, as described in Meiner's piece, which aim to expand the market for LTCI to the middle-class population that is most likely to exhaust its resources on LTC expenditures, eventually qualifying for coverage through the Medicaid program. Some argue that one of the reasons that take-up for private LTCI is so poor is because insurers focus on wealthy individuals, who are more likely to purchase LTC insurance and favor more comprehensive (and expensive) benefit packages that aim to cover most nursing home costs (Feder, Komisar, & Friedland, 2007; LifePlans, Inc., 2007). The Partnership Program was one effort to expand the market for LTCI by permitting individuals who purchased a modest private plan to protect substantially more assets before qualifying for Medicaid (otherwise, they must exhaust most private assets first). The more extensive the coverage purchased, the more a LTC Partnership Program participant could save. Following the 2005 Deficit Reduction Act (DRA), which moved the program from demonstration status to a regular part of the Medicaid program, the number of participating states expanded from four to 40, and the number of policies held expanded from about 400,000 to 520,000 (Long-Term Care Partnership Program, 2011). This slow take-up has caused some to question whether asset protection is in fact a motivating factor for LTCI purchase; Wiener (2010) also notes that premiums for Partnership products remain high–about two-thirds pay over $1,500 annually.

In contrast to the Partnership Programs' limited reach, CLASS, discussed by Meiners, Weissert, and Wiener, represented a rare ambitious step with respect to LTC policy – although it is widely agreed to be deeply problematic (as all the authors point out, Wiener most extensively). CLASS aimed to offer only partial coverage for the cost of LTC, by providing a low-level benefit averaging $50 per day, which was not intended to cover the full costs of nursing home care. Debates over the value of this legislation centered on the extent to which it would have made progress toward solving the nation's LTC financing problem.

Government programs to protect citizens against the risk of LTC could either: (1) focus on covering catastrophic costs (that is, the cost of extended nursing home care), as Weissert argues, or (2) focus on mitigating the financial impact of ongoing costs in whatever setting, institutional or non-institutional (what Meiners calls "front-end risk"), while keeping Medicaid in place as a backstop in the case of catastrophic expenses. Given Medicaid's now-extensive role in providing home- and community-based services, adoption of the latter option—that is, CLASS—could in fact play an important role in reducing dependence on the Medicaid program and its associated expenditures. In 2008, Medicaid paid around $12,500 toward the average per capita costs of aged and disabled individuals served through home- and community-based programs, an amount that compares favorably to the size of the expected CLASS benefit. Indeed, the CLASS approach is the one typically followed by developed nations that offer public insurance coverage for LTC costs (although other nation's make participation mandatory whereas participation would have been voluntary in CLASS) (Colombo, Llena-Nozal, Mercier & Tjadens, 2011). Such a path allows for supplementation via means-tested public programs or via the private market, as in France, for example, where 30% of those 60 or older purchase private LTCI (Nadash, Doty, Mahoney, & von Schwanenflugel, 2012).

Weissert, on the other hand, argues that the risk of needing extended care in nursing homes is the critical factor that government needs to address through the adoption of an insurance program such as CLASS. He notes an increasing divergence in the populations served in nursing home and community-based settings–although it should be noted that state and federal policies, as well as financial incentives, dictate that more and more people requiring a nursing home level of care are being served in the community (Cheek et al., 2012, Kaiser, 2011). The data he relies on for lifetime risk of nursing home stay date from Murtaugh et al's 1997 paper (using data from 1995); more recent figures suggest that lifetime risk of nursing home placement has dropped, from 40% in 1995 to 35% 2005 (Kemper, Komisar & Alexcih, 2006). What is more these latter data show that 18% of those 65 or older have a stay of 1 year or more, with 5% having a stay of 5 years or more. While the overall risk appears to have dropped only somewhat, the risk of a long stay has dropped considerably–Weissert cites a 20% risk of a 5 year stay, which contrasts considerably with the 5% risk found by Kemper et al.

It seems likely that more recent figures would show an even lower risk of nursing home use—particularly, of extended nursing home stays—due to the market-driven expansion of assisted living facilities and the policy-driven shift of individuals out of nursing homes to home- and community-based settings wherever possible. This has been part of a gradual shift, more acute in some states than in others (see Table 1 in the Harrington piece), reinforced by the 1999 *Olmstead v. L.C.* decision of the U.S. Supreme Court, which placed a burden on states to serve individuals in the least restrictive environment possible. But Increased reliance on home- and community-based services also has to do with a cultural and political shift toward supporting aging in place, and awareness of the financial implications of relying on nursing homes as a primary site of LTC delivery. Thus, individuals who might previously have been placed in nursing homes are now being served in community-based settings.

The Harrington paper discusses how this trend is being continued through the ACA, which extends a variety of federal initiatives to move people out of nursing homes and into non-institutional settings. The most significant of these is the Community First option, which creates significant incentives for states to expand access to home- and community-based services. However, its potential is considerably dampened by the current financial and political climate, which makes states reluctant to adopt additional responsibilities, no matter how favorable the incentive, for fear of incurring liabilities that they may not be in a position to meet. Another change is the technical fixes to the home- and community-based services state plan option, which should provide states with the opportunity to create administrative efficiencies through the consolidation of existing waivers into a single program. Prior to the ACA, much state innovation in home- and community-based services has been through the waive mechanism, whereby states apply for waivers (of the standard Medicaid benefit program) from the federal government to offer supplementary services to specific populations (see Thompson & Burke, 2008 for an overview), creating, in some states, a confusing and inefficient array of service programs; the ACA option should considerably simplify that. Observers seem to be less optimistic about the potential of the third change, the State Balancing Incentive Program, given that few states are likely to be up to the challenge of instituting its requirements in the current environment– requirements that must be met within six months of the application date, such as establishing a single entry point system and implementing a statewide tool for determining eligibility for home- and community-based services. Although all of these initiatives are welcome, they are dependent on state initiative and, once again, represent only partial and incremental approaches to addressing the need for LTC.

Of course, Weissert is quite right about the devastating financial consequences of extended nursing home stays for those who do require them. But is it government's role to protect against this risk for the whole population, or for the poor only (as the current system does, via the Medicaid program)? Meiners raises the provocative possibility that government might offer people a choice of options under the CLASS program, allowing people to choose the level of protection they would like. However, this kind of choice in insurance options always raises the specter of risk segmentation (i.e., adverse selection); moreover, such a diversity of options might be of interest to well-informed consumers only and may in fact deter less sophisticated purchasers from participating. Weighing up these alternate plan designs requires a level of understanding both of the true risks that most of us face, as well as of insurance concepts such as deductibles and inflation protection that may be obscure to the population it is most important to reach.

And the breadth of coverage is only one of the controversial issues raised by CLASS. Wiener discusses a broad range of such issues, raising the question of whether any form of voluntary insurance program can succeed, given the clear risk selection issues raised by a LTCI program, and whether there are mechanisms that might mitigate these, including, perhaps, risk-adjusted payments from government (or other forms of re-insurance), to even out selection issues; sophisticated marketing to ensure take-up or cross-subsidies from general revenue or other public programs, to ensure the affordability of premiums. Wiener points out other important issues, too, such as who should be covered (people who are long-term-disabled or who have no work history?), for how long (lifetime coverage?), and what form the benefit should take (cash?). And while it is tempting to evaluate these questions on purely technical grounds—that is, whether such a program can be made to work financially—it is clear that, to develop a meaningful LTC insurance program that commands broad public support, we also need to consider a far wider range of questions on what role private LTCI should play, what role the government should play through a public LTC insurance such as CLASS, and what role the government should play through a means-tested safety-net program such as Medicaid.

While the stalled CLASS initiative addressed LTC financing, other parts of the ACA address a variety of other issues in LTC: most notably, cost and quality. Efforts to coordinate care are discussed in the Grabowski piece. Such efforts target the sickest and most expensive older people–those who are dually eligible for Medicare and Medicaid, most often due to their need for LTC. They also typically focus on improving coordination of the complex array of services these people receive, and integrating Medicare, Medicaid, and other financing, to allow organizations to better manage their services.

With the exception of the Independence at Home Initiative, however, the ACA focuses either on financing or delivery reform rather than tackling both together, as current programs such as the Program for Inclusive Care for the Elderly and Minnesota Senior Health Options do. Grabowski therefore raises concerns about the potential for the ACA to achieve better results than prior efforts have–concerns echoed in recent Congressional Budget Office reports summarizing the research on Medicare disease management and care coordination programs, which found that on average the programs did not recoup their costs, and on value-based payment experiments in the Medicare program, where results were "mixed", with only one program achieving savings (Nelson, 2012a, 2012b). There appears to be agreement that, while the ACA may prove effective in improving coordination, genuine cost savings and more ambitious reform will depend on structural changes that are currently not likely.

Despite the shift toward home- and community-based services described by Harrington, nursing homes remain an important component of the LTC system. Quality in this area has always been an issue, and has been addressed sporadically over the years, most comprehensively through the Omnibus Budget Reconciliation Act (OBRA) of 1987, which introduced important oversight and resident protection measures. However, enforcement of the OBRA standards has been an ongoing issue (Hawes, et al. references the many U.S. General Accountability Office reports, spanning 1999 through 2009, recounting continuing problems in this area). Thus it is likely that the impact of government on nursing home quality will depend largely on the extent to which Congress invests in enforcement of current law and the regulations that support it. The ACA provisions in this area, by contrast, continue incremental trends toward pay-for-performance and increased transparency (via reporting requirements and the Nursing Home Compare website) that have been established already. Once again, the lack of a more comprehensive approach to nursing home quality reveals LTC policy as the poor stepchild of health care policy development in the U.S.

Of course, to implement the changes discussed by Grabowski and Hawes, there will need to be well-trained individuals ready to take on the tasks that the various quality improvement approaches and new service models included within the ACA bring. Robyn Stone's piece welcomes the advances made under the ACA in addressing some key issues in the LTC workforce—but points out that the legislation fails to adequately address the critical shortages in nearly every class of provider—but most especially, direct care workers—trained to deal with the challenges posed by an aging society. Moreover, the lack of Congressional appropriations thus far, as well as the limited allocation under the legislation for the ACA provisions in this area, bodes ill for their ability to have an impact on workforce readiness. Still, the ACA is the first major piece of federal legislation that acknowledges and addresses these workforce deficiencies in a coherent way and, in that respect, does represent an important step forward.

A further question is the overall impact of the ACA on older people generally. Moon outlines the various ACA provisions affecting Medicare beneficiaries. On the plus side, they will see improvements in coverage for preventive treatments and expanded coverage for prescription drug costs (to list just a few). On the minus side, cuts in payments for Medicare providers, reduced payment for Medicare Advantage plans, and restrictions on access to specific services, such as home health, may have negative impacts on access to services. Although ACA efforts that address system-wide cost issues, such as the Patient-Centered Outcomes Research Institute (which aims to identify effective treatments) and the Independent Payment Advisory Board (which aims to identify ways to restrain Medicare costs), may also end up benefiting older people more generally, like so much about the ACA, the overall impact of these provisions will depend vitally on how they are implemented and on whether the health care system as a whole is indeed fundamentally reshaped by the law. We must also be alert for future legislation proposing even more significant re-shaping of the healthcare system, such as the various premium support proposals currently under discussion for the Medicare program (vouchering), as well as other proposals for eligibility changes and steeper income adjustments.

The potential for the ACA to constitute an important step forward for the health and LTC of older people is significantly constrained by a number of factors. The current political and economic environment is probably the most serious of these, making it difficult for policymakers to advance initiatives that can be cast as spending increases—particularly spending on older people—at either the federal- or state-levels. Thus legislative provisions that are consistent with ongoing trends in health and LTC are likely to receive the least resistance. However, unless Congress follows up with the appropriations, enforcement, and regulations necessary to implement these provisions, the advances promulgated in LTC service delivery and regulation are likely to prove disappointing.

REFERENCES

Ahlstrom, A., Tumlinson, A., Lambrew, J. (2004). *Linking Reverse Mortgages and Long-Term Care Insurance*. Washington, DC: The Brookings Institution. Retrieved from http://www.brookings.edu/~/media/Files/rc/papers/2004/03useconomics_ahlstrom/20040317.pdf

Cheek, M., Roherty, M., Finnan, L., Cho, E., Walls, J., Gifford, K., Fox-Grage, W., Ujvari, K. (2012). *On the Verge: The Transformation of Long-Term Services and Supports*. Washington, DC: AARP Public Policy Institute. Retrieved from http://www.aarp.org/content/dam/aarp/research/public_policy_institute/ltc/2012/On-the-Verge-The-Transformation-of-Long-Term-Services-and-Supports-Report-AARP-ppi-ltc.pdf

Colombo, F. Llena-Nozal, A., Mercier, J., Tjadens, F. (2011). *Help Wanted? Providing and Paying for Long-Term Care, OECD Health Policy Studies*. OECD Publishing. Retrieved from http://www.oecd-ilibrary.org/social-issues-migration-health/help-wanted_9789264097759-en

Department of Health and Human Services (DHHS) (October 14, 2011). *Secretary Sebelius' Letter to Congress about CLASS*. Retrieved from http://www.hhs.gov/secretary/letter10142011.html

Feder, J., Komisar, H.L., Friedland, R.B. (2007). *Long-term care financing: Policy options for the future*. Washington, DC: Health Policy Institute, Georgetown University. Retrieved from http://ltc.georgetown.edu/forum/ltcfinalpaper061107.pdf

Gleckman, H. (January, 26, 2010). Creation of federal long-term care program on hold. *Forbes*. Retrieved from http://www.forbes.com/sites/howardgleckman/2011/09/26/creation-of-federal-long-term-care-program-on-hold/

Kaiser Family Foundation, (2011). *Medicaid Home and Community-Based Service Programs: Data Update*. Washington, DC: Kaiser. Retrieved from http://www.kff.org/medicaid/upload/7720-05.pdf

Kemper, P., Komisar, H.L., & Alexcih, L. (2006). Long-term care over an uncertain future: What can current retirees expect? *Inquiry*. 42, 335—350.

LifePlans, Inc. (2007). *Who Buys Long-Term Care Insurance? A 15-year Study of Buyers and Non-Buyers, 1990-2005*. America's Health Insurance Plans. Retrieved from http://www.ahipresearch.org/PDFs/LTC_Buyers_Guide.pdf

Long-Term Care Partnership Program. (2011). *DRA Partnership Reports*. Retrieved from http://w2.dehpg.net/LTCPartnership/Reports.aspx.

Marmor, T.R. 2000. *The politics of Medicare.* (2nd Edition). New York: Aldine de Gruyter.

Mature Market Institute (2009, September). *MetLife Long-Term Care IQ: Long-Term Care IQ: Removing Myths, Reinforcing Realities.* Westport, CT: Author. Retrieved from http://www.metlife.com/assets/cao/mmi/publications/consumer/long-term-care-essentials/mmi-long-term-care-iq-removing-myths-survey.pdf

Mature Market Institute (2011, October). *The 2011 MetLife Market Survey of Nursing Home, Assisted Living, Adult Day Services, and Home Care Costs.* Westport, CT: Author. Retrieved from www.metlife.com/assets/cao/mmi/publications/studies/2011/mmi-market-survey-nursing-home-assisted-living-adult-day-services-costs.pdf

Moses, S.A. (2005). *Aging America's Achilles' Heel: Medicaid Long-Term Care. Policy Analysis 549.* Washington, DC: The Cato Institute. Retrieved from http://www.cato.org/pubs/pas/pa549.pdf

Murtaugh, C.M., Kemper, P.. Spillman, B.C., & Carlson, B.L.. (1997). The amount, distribution, and timing of lifetime nursing Home Use. *Medical Care,* 35(3), 204—218.

Murtaugh, C.M., Spillman, B.C., & Warshawsky, M.J. (2001). In sickness and in health: An annuity approach to financing long-term care and retirement income. *The Journal of Risk and Insurance,* 68(2), 225—254.

Nadash, P., Doty, P., Mahoney, K., & von Schwanenflugel, M. (2012). European long term care programs: Lessons for CLASS? *Health Services Research,* 47(1), 309—328.

Nelson, L. (January 2012a). *Lessons from Medicare's Demonstration Projects on Disease Management and Care Coordination. Working Paper 2012-01.* Washington, DC: Congressional Budget Office. Retrieved from http://www.cbo.gov/sites/default/files/cbofiles/attachments/WP2012-01_Nelson_Medicare_DMCC_Demonstrations.pdf

Nelson, L. (January 2012b). *Lessons from Medicare's Demonstration Projects on Value-Based Payment. Working Paper 2012-02.* Washington, DC: Congressional Budget Office. Retrieved from http://www.cbo.gov/sites/default/files/cbofiles/attachments/WP2012-02_Nelson_Medicare_VBP_Demonstrations.pdf

Ogden, L.L. & Adams, K. (2008). Poorhouse to warehouse: institutional long-term care in the United States, *Publius,* 39(1), 138—163.

Smith, D.B. & Feng, Z. (2010). The accumulated challenges of long-term care. *Health Affairs,* 29(1), 29—34.

Thompson, F.J. & Burke, C. (2008). Federalism by waiver: Medicaid and the transformation of long-term care. *Publius,* 39(1), 22—46.

Tuohy, C.H. (2011). American health reform in comparative perspective: Big bang, blueprint, or mosaic? *Journal of Health Politics, Policy and Law,* 36(3), 571—576.

Wiener J.M. (2010). *Long-Term Care in Hawaii: Issues and Options.* Presentation to the Hawaii Long-Term Care Commission, March 12, 2010.

Yee, D. (2001). Long-term care policy and financing as a public or private matter in the United States. *Journal of Aging & Social Policy,* 13(2/3), 35—51.

Index

ROUTLEDGE

Related titles from Routledge

Family Support and Family Caregiving across Disabilities

Edited by George H.S. Singer, David E. Biegel and Patricia Conway

Family members provide the majority of care for individuals with disabilities in the United States. Recognition is growing that family caregiving deserves and may require societal support, and evidence-based practices have been established for reducing stress associated with caregiving. Despite the substantial research literature on family support that has developed, researchers, advocates and professionals have often worked in separate categorical domains such as family support for caregiving for the frail elderly, for individuals with mental illness, or for people with development disabilities.

This book addresses this significant limitation through cross-categorical and lifespan analyses of family support and family caregiving from the perspectives of theory and conceptual frameworks, empirical research and frameworks and recommendations for improvements in public policy. It also examines children with disabilities, children with autism, adults with schizophrenia, and individuals with cancer across the life cycle.

This book was published as a two-part special issue in the *Journal of Family Social Work*.

August 2011: 246 x 174: 216pp
Hb: 978-0-415-68268-8
£80 / $125

Available from all good bookshops